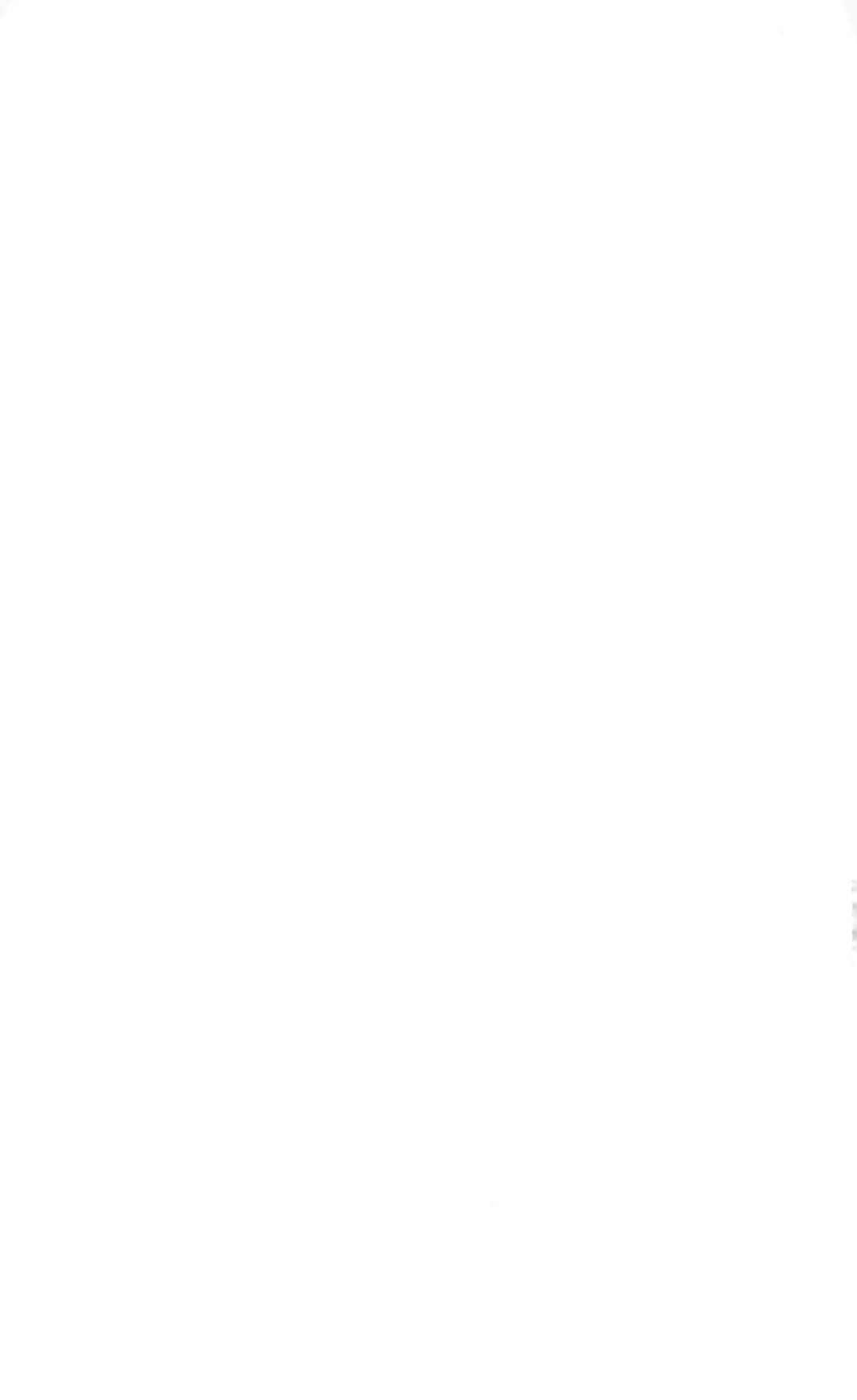

Orthopantomography

Ignazio Pandolfo • Silvio Mazziotti

Orthopantomography

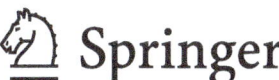 Springer

Authors
Ignazio Pandolfo
Department of Radiological Sciences
University of Messina
Messina
Italy

Silvio Mazziotti
Department of Radiological Sciences
University of Messina
Messina
Italy

Contributing Authors
Tommaso D'Angelo M.D.
Department of Radiological Sciences
University of Messina
Messina
Italy

Sergio Racchiusa M.D.
Department of Radiological Sciences
University of Messina
Messina
Italy

ISBN 978-88-470-5288-8   ISBN 978-88-470-5289-5   (eBook)
DOI 10.1007/978-88-470-5289-5
Springer Milan Heidelberg New York Dordrecht London

Library of Congress Control Number: 2013933871

Printed on acid-free paper

Springer is part of Springer Science+Business Media (www.springer.com)

Contents

Part I

Technique and Normal Anatomy

Orthopantomography (OPT) is the most widespread radiographic investigation carried out today. It represents an extraoral study technique in which both revelation system and radiogenic source are external to the oral cavity.

OPT is a radiologic examination which allows to accurately plan odontoiatric treatment in a remarkable number of cases. Indeed, the methodology is able to provide complex data on the masticatory apparatus and the surrounding structures allowing the evaluation of normal anatomy and the majority of pathological conditions. **Orthopantomography** is also called **panoramic radiography of dental arches**. The term orthopantomography comes from the Greek words: ορθος ("ortós": orthogonal) = radiant beam perpendicular to the teeth major axis, παν ("pán": all) = global vision of both arches and τομος ("tómos": cut, section) = radiological technique able to generate section images (**tomography**), a methodology known in traditional radiology also as **stratigraphy**. It exploits the cancellation principle through the **kinetic blur** of the structures beyond the interest area.

Therefore, OPT is a radiographic technique, allowing to achieve panoramic radiograms which are able to demonstrate anatomical complex structures. It includes not only dental arches but also paranasal sinuses, superior and inferior maxillaries and temporomandibular joints.

Consequently, panoramic radiography's hardest challenge is to transfer the aforementioned anatomical structures into a bidimensional radiological image. Those images are characterised by correct parameters of exposition and by the minor rate of structure superimposition and geometrical distortion. There is no doubt that this goal is not easy to achieve when considering the extreme variability of patient's morphology and structure thickness taken into examination. Moreover, innumerable individual differences among the whole population have to be considered. OPT is based on the simultaneous employment and integration of two basic principles which derive from traditional radiology: **tomography** and **fissure radiography**.

Tomography is a technique which consists in a synchronous and integral movement, occurring in opposed directions, of radiogenic source (radiogenic tube) and

I. Pandolfo, S. Mazziotti, *Orthopantomography*,
DOI 10.1007/978-88-470-5289-5_1, © Springer-Verlag Italia 2013

revelation system (radiographic film or digital detector), around a mechanically fixed point, called rotation fulcrum, which identifies the interest area (**tomographic plane**).

The tube detection system movement gives rise to structures' cancellation beyond the interest area (both in front and behind). This is the result of **kinetic blur** or movement blur optical phenomenon. In OPT, such movement is realised with arch trajectories at about 200–240° (Fig. 1.1).

As a consequence of what was aforementioned, a clear representation of all anatomical structures included in the tomographic plane is realised. The representation is radiographically optimal, as it is 'in focus'. This is possible as the system **rotation fulcrum** corresponds to the structure of interest, which, during the tube detector translation movement, appears optically still. Thereby, they are better radiologically representable than what is situated beyond the tomographic plane, which will be blurred and therefore deleted. The cancellation phenomenon turns out to be only partial. Indeed some structures, even if out of the interest plane, can interfere with the final image, generating the so-called parasite images or images of transport. This is due to their high density or radiolucency and/or their close anatomical contiguity to the area of interest.

It is more to say that, in linear tomography, the thickness layer varies depending on the 'oscillation angle' (major angles generate thinner layers whereas minor angles determine thicker layers).

The principle of tomography applied in OPT is obviously adapted to the need of representing curvilinear morphology structures, such as dental arcades. Indeed, OPT mainly exploits, not only one rotation fulcrum (as it happens in normal linear tomography) but three rotation fulcrums (one for each lateral arcade and one for the central elements' representation). Angular movement of the tomographic system creates a minor angle to represent lateral arcades (characterised by major thickness), while it performs a major angle to represent frontal elements (which present minor thickness).

Thereby, this technical peculiarity allows to adapt the thickness of the tomographic plane to different thicknesses which characterise maxillaries' various portions.

Therefore, the tomographic movement articulated in three fulcrums generates a section plane with variable thickness which can be quantified in about 15–16 mm for lateral sectors analysis and about 8–9 mm for the study of thinner structures characterising the frontal part of the dental arcades (Fig. 1.2).

Tomographic systems with **variable geometry rotation fulcrum** are the most technologically advanced pieces of equipment, performing well in image quality. They do not employ fixed rotation fulcrums, but realise a unique fulcrum continuous variation along a prefixed elliptical trajectory.

Those tools allow to operate, according to the case, using different elliptical trajectories which are adaptable in different needs (paediatric age, jaws' malformations, etc.)

OPT system rotation time, and therefore image acquisition time (independently on the type of technology used), varies from about 15 to 20 s.

Fissure radiography or scanography represents the other OPT technical peculiarity.

It entails the use of a **fissure collimator** (from which fissure radiography takes its name) aiming at eliminating the radiation beam oblique component.

This artifice reduces the photon beam into a thin sheet, hitting selectively the single dental alveolus elements. The relative image is gradually impressed on a thin layer of the film. Such image is deprived of any deformations and has a minor diffuse radiation.

This procedure is possible thanks to the tube and the collimator synchronical movement. As a consequence, the revelation system (radiographic film or digital plate) is progressively impressed.

The digital revelation system or radiographic cassette, beyond the already translation movement described above, will obviously have a running capacity articulated in autonomous micromovements. As a consequence, always different points of the revelation system detection plane will be exposed to the photon layer.

Methodology

The following paragraph generically illustrates technical and methodological problems, as it is impossible to fully analyse the peculiarity of the numerous equipment typology present in the market today.

A particular preparation of the patient is not requested in order to carry out a correct OPT examination; however, it is absolutely necessary to remove all that can disturb the final image (earrings, dentures, hairpins, piercing, etc.)

A fundamental methodological artifice entails the insertion of a removable clamp between the central incisors margin. This allows the elements of superior and inferior arcades to be placed in the same line and in vertical position. As a consequence, they completely fall into the tomographic plane, giving rise to an optimal radiological representation.

It is very clear that excessive inclination of incisive elements or errors in the head collocation make those dental elements fall entirely or partially out of the tomographic plane. This gives rise to a deficient representation of the apical region or the crown and sometimes of both structures (Figs. 1.3, 1.4, and 1.5).

Moreover, it will be necessary to place the head on a provided base or **submental support plane**, to accurately regulate the height of the cassette support and establish the head position.

The submental support is obviously essential for edentulous patients in whom the removable clamp cannot be used. Three linear luminous reference lines regulate head positioning. The first line is in the horizontal plane and has to be aligned with the Frankfurt plane. Another line is vertical, in order to identify the midsagittal plane. The latter, which is vertical too, is situated on the lateral surface of the patient's face, which must coincide with the canine–incisive region. Finally, such line will determine the position of the frontal group elements in respect to the tomographic plane (Fig. 1.6a, b).

This coincidence will be obviously realised, case by case, with appropriate linear adjustments of the position and the removable clamp.

It is fundamental to invite the patient to close his lips and to push his tongue against the hard palate (in order to eliminate the artefacts deriving from aerial content which is comprised between the tongue and the palatal arch).

In addition, it will be appropriate to explain the examination modality and length to the patient, inviting him to stand still for the whole time.

It is not advisable to use proteximetric devices for the neck, as their artefacts can sometimes cause the examination repetition. Finally, in order to have a correct OPT execution, it will be necessary for the patient to catch the apposite support with his hands, to bring together his feet in front of the body and to keep the incisors attached to the clamp.

This posture (also called the **position of the 'water skier'**) aims at withdrawing the cervical spine, moving it away from the rotation fulcrum and the detection plane. This artifice determines the minimisation of the noise, due to the transport shadow of the cervical spine on the final radiogram (Fig. 1.7).

Errors and Artefacts in OPT

As OPT is a complex methodology, it suffers from numerous limitations which can interfere with the diagnosis. Those limitations can be summarised as follows:
1. Operator's errors
2. Patient's artefacts
3. Artefacts generated by machine intrinsic characteristics or by its malfunctioning.

It is of extreme importance for the radiologist to be able to recognise artefact nature and origin, in order to get their entire or partial elimination (when possible).

Several are the errors and the consequent artefacts which can be found in OPT. They can be classified into four categories:
1. **Patient preparation errors** (Fig. 1.8)
2. **Patient instruction errors** (Fig. 1.9)
3. **Cassette collocation errors** (Figs. 1.10, 1.11, and 1.12)
4. **Patient positioning errors** (Fig. 1.13)

Patient Preparation Errors

Such category includes the most banal errors, such as performing the radiogram with removable dental prosthesis, earrings, piercing, necklaces, etc. All these objects, due to their high opacity, can interfere with the structures in exam, causing parasite images of transport (Fig. 1.8).

Patient Instruction Errors

Patient's instruction is a crucial element for the investigation success. The technician has to clearly transfer all the information in order to obtain a correct radiographic procedure.

Indeed, it is recommendable to remind the patient to stand absolutely still and to give him instructions about the correct apposition of the tongue to the hard palate. This operation must be verified in advance. Failure to comply with this requirement may cause movement artefacts and/or a radiolucent area in the central region of the superior maxilla. That will make the radiogram difficult and even impossible to evaluate (Fig. 1.9).

Unfortunately, it must be underlined that those artifices cannot always be applied to paediatric age patients or to adults with a poor cognitive level (psychiatric pathologies, advanced age, etc.). As a consequence, there will be a deficiency in the radiological result.

It is considered appropriate for the radiologist to report the aforementioned insuperable difficulties, in order to illustrate the causes of a poor-quality image.

Cassette Location Errors

Concerning those kinds of errors, it is to say that they mainly depend on the type of the available equipment; therefore, they cannot be summarised in a global perspective.

Cassette and/or cassette support location is one of the most common mistake. It is often placed too below or above the mandible (Fig. 1.10).

The wrong location of the cassette and/or cassette support can generate an abnormal contact with the patient's shoulder. Such contact can interfere with the system translation movement, blocking and/or slowing it down.

As a consequence an overexposure band corresponding to the absorption profile can occur. At such level temporary arrest and/or a slowing down of the system movement can cause in fact the overexposure of the detection plane (Fig. 1.11a, b).

Obviously, a similar artefact can depend also on the patient's particular physical conformation (short neck, shoulder prominence, etc.). Conversely, underexposure bands can be correlated to a malfunctioning of the system, which generates a translation speed increase at a given fissure level. Consequently, such level will be characterised by minor irradiation of the detection system (Fig. 1.12a, b).

In relation to what stated before, the entity and the frequency of the above-mentioned **overexposure and underexposure artefacts** are significantly influenced by the good functioning of the **automatic exposure system**. The automatic exposure system, as is known, is able to regulate and optimise photon emission, depending on the blackening of the detection system.

Patient Positioning Errors

It has already been described which is the correct patient's positioning, both on the axial and sagittal planes.

The positioning on the axial plane must accomplish with the fundamental goal of putting in parallel the hard palate (identified with the line which corresponds to the Frankfurt plane) and the horizontal plane. Thus, they will coincide perfectly.

This coincidence generates radiographic representation of the hard palate as a thin radiopaque streak (Fig. 1.13).

The inclination error of the hard palate, in respect to the horizontal plane, can be both in positive (in head hyperextension) (Fig. 1.14) and in negative (in hyperflexion) (Fig. 1.15).

The wrong inclination of the hard palate generates a radiopaque band which, if projected downwards, can interfere with the visibility of the teeth apices of the superior arches (Fig. 1.16).

On the contrary, positive wrong inclination will give rise to images of transport. This is due to the unwanted structure (e.g. the soft palate) approach to the tomographic plane (Fig. 1.17).

Moreover, such mistake will cause a back movement of the inferior incisors, which consequently will come out from the tomographic plane.

Finally, it is to say that the aforementioned errors of head inclination can influence the partial intrusion of other structures in the tomographic plane. These structures, because of their parasite images, can damage the radiogram quality.

In regard to this problem, nasal pyramid image of transport is illustrative. It can generate difficulty in the analysis of the superior incisive bundle elements and/or it can create fake images in the apical region of the aforementioned elements (Fig. 1.18a, b).

Moreover, the patient's positioning of the 'water skier', as already explained, has the goal of determinating cervical spine withdrawal with respect to the tomographic plane.

Indeed, the back position of the head and the body advance will cause cervical spine withdrawal and its obliquity on the sagittal plane with a front-back and a bottom-up orientation. Conversely, the lack of this methodological artifice determines a completely opposite attitude of the cervical spine, involving it in the image formation. It follows that a thick and median opaque band will appear, impeding incisive element analysis (Figs. 1.19a, b and 1.20a, b).

The already mentioned incisors' wrong positioning in the clamp has to be included among positioning errors. Its consequence is a nonlinear placement of superior and/or inferior incisors in respect to the tomographic plane.

Finally, it has to be remembered that edentulism of the incisors makes mandatory the acquisition without clamp, using the submental support only. As a consequence, poor images are obtained.

Furthermore, acquisition without clamp, as integrative technique of the standard examination, is also possible in the presence of particular anatomical situations.

Indeed, this methodological artifice can sometimes contribute to improve the visibility of teeth apices and interdental spaces (Fig. 1.21).

Geometrical Enlargement in OPT

As all the radiological investigations, dental panoramic is influenced by physic laws which rule the projective geometrical enlargement. Basically, this phenomenon is inversely proportional to the distance between the tube and the detection plane (which in OPT is fixed, therefore unchangeable). On the other hand, it is directly proportional to the distance which exists between the object and the detection plane, which, conversely, can vary both for positioning errors and for the patient's morphological features.

Very briefly, the distance increase between the object and the detection plane will cause a dimensional increment of the object radiological representation.

However, as in OPT, the aforementioned distance is never equal to zero, the panoramic radiogram will always be loaded by a certain enlargement which is quantifiable in about 15–20 %. It varies according to the equipment brand and type.

The radiological enlargement in OPT is characterised by two components: **horizontal enlargement** and **vertical enlargement** (the latter is obviously of major importance for implant surgery planning).

Taking into account those considerations, measurements obtained in OPT turn out to be unreliable and not suitable for the preimplant planning.

In order to avoid the aforementioned problem, dedicated software programs have been proposed in digital OPT. They are able to elaborate OPT digital data providing the image representation of the dental arcades. Such representation turns out to be faithful to the original dimensions (**enlargement scale 1 to 1**).

The employment of steel wires of known dimensions is another methodological artifice (radiopaque spheres or **dime**, generally with a diameter of 0.5 cm). They are installed in apposite supports (**bite**) and worn by the patient at the moment of the examination.

Such steel wires allow the calculation of the enlargement percentage by mathematical extrapolation.

The aforementioned systems, even if theoretically efficient in the dimensional evaluation, present at least two weak points.

The first one is represented by the fact that, in the given subject, OPT radiographic enlargement may not be equal and homogeneous in all the maxillary districts.

The second one comes from the consideration that, also in the presence of trustful measurements, the radiological image is characterised by a lack of tridimensional information. Therefore, it does not allow to evaluate structure thickness and their space disposition (e.g. the alveolar ridge inclination).

Dimensional distortions can also occur as a consequence of the errors in the patient's head positioning.

The artefact introduced by the error is absolutely peculiar and distinctive. It consists on positioning the patient's head too far or too close to the detection plane.

Such methodological error generates panoramic images, characterised by a geometrical distortion which can cause difficulties in the radiogram analysis (Fig. 1.22a, b).

Any error related to head positioning in respect to the sagittal plane can cause enlargement and geometry distortions. Such errors entail head rotation on its longitudinal axis, both in clockwise and anticlockwise direction (Fig. 1.23).

Because of such positioning errors, half of the masticatory apparatus which is farther from the cassette will appear geometrically enlarged, both in horizontal and vertical direction (Fig. 1.24). Therefore, the nearest half will appear smaller (Fig. 1.25).

The so-called interproximal superimposition artefact which, as known, can make impossible the interdental space evaluation takes its own genesis in the distortion introduced by the geometrical enlargement phenomenon.

Indeed, dental elements, set far from the detection plane (e.g. in lingual position), will suffer from a significant geometrical enlargement. As a consequence, their image will be geometrically superimposed on the adjacent elements which are not enlarged. Thus, they will obliterate the interdental space with their opacity (Fig. 1.26).

Finally, as explained above, it is possible to state that some errors, depending on simple negligence in the execution of the examination, can be easily avoidable.

Conversely, artefacts originating from the patient's collaborative capacity or from his body morphology can be basically ineliminable.

In regard to this, it must be mentioned the noise generated by transport shadows such as hyoid bone, soft palate and epiglottis. Even if these shadows can be caused by the patient's positioning errors, they are, most of the times, related to morphology and neck dimensions.

Moreover, not all the aforementioned artefacts are able to compromise the diagnosis in significant way. Therefore, it is not always necessary to repeat the examination.

Finally, the introduction of digital technology currently consents to further reduce the necessity of additional radiographic examinations.

In addition, digital technology allows to evaluate the image post-processing (enlargement observation, positive–negative inversion, modification of the blackening through the regulation of the data representation). Those techniques allow to reduce the need of extra radiographic examinations.

Furthermore, image digitalisation has eliminated all those artefacts which are typical of the analogic film, such as the ones related to chemical treatment, storage problems and/or manipulation (electrical discharge, fingerprints, etc.).

Image Gallery

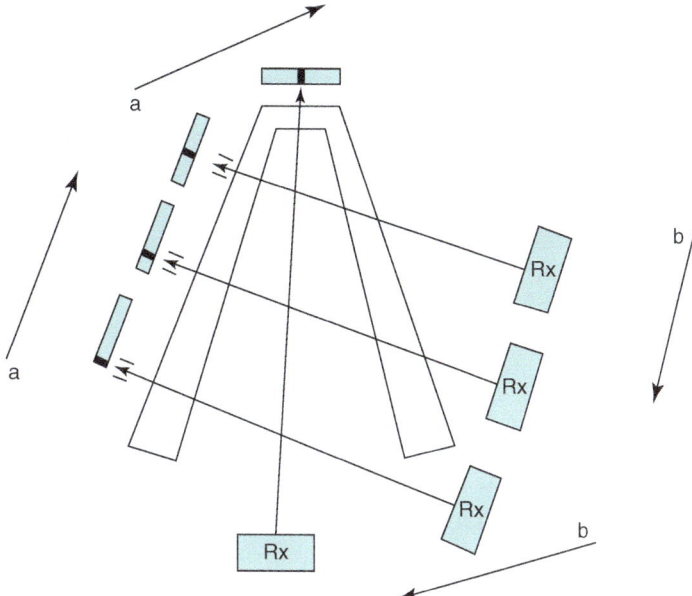

Fig. 1.1 Diagram illustrating the stratigraphic translation of the tube detection system in OPT. The *arrows* marked *a* indicate the movement of the revelation system; *arrows* marked *b* indicate the tube movement which occurs in opposed direction. The diagram represents the acquisition of a single hemi-arcade and the frontal region. *Rx* X-ray source

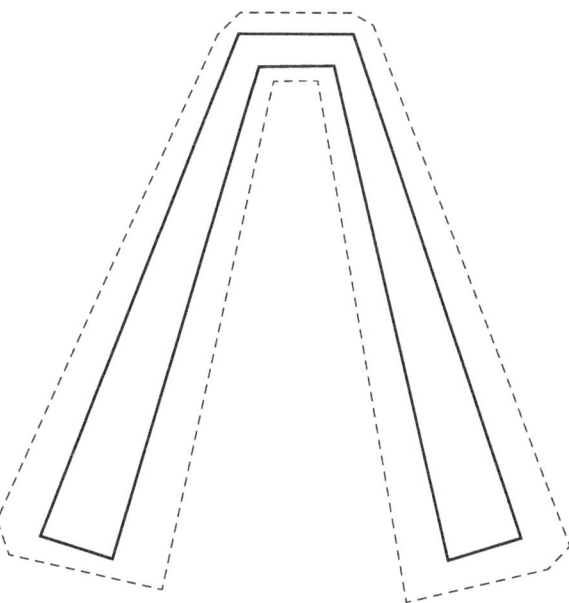

Fig. 1.2 The *dashed line* indicates the layer thickness which is thicker at the level of the lateral maxillaries and thinner in the region of the frontal elements

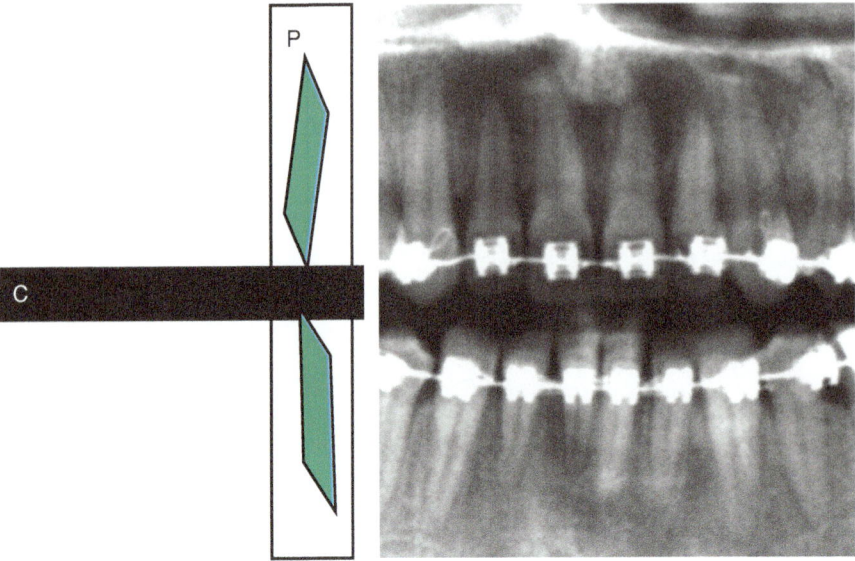

Fig. 1.3 The image shows the correct position of the incisive elements in the tomographic plane. The radiographic representation shows that the incisive elements are perfectly in focus, both at apical and crown level. *P* plane, *C* clamp

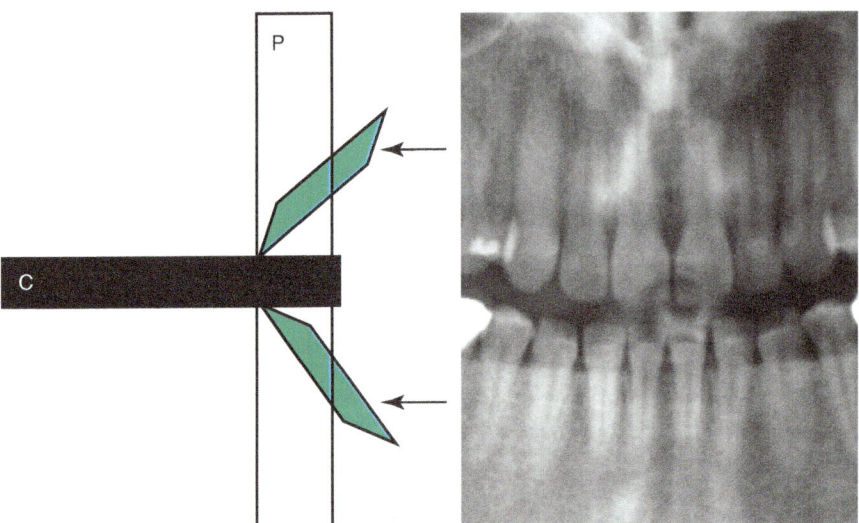

Fig. 1.4 Excessive inclination of the incisive elements makes the apices (represented by *arrows*) fall out of the tomographic plane. Therefore, they appear scarcely defined as they are not 'in focus'. This is visible in the radiographic representation. *P* plane, *C* clamp

Fig. 1.5 A major inclination of the incisive elements or the wrong positioning of the tomographic plane can give rise to a deficient representation of the incisive elements' apical region and crown (the incisive elements are indicated by *arrows*) *P* plane, *C* clamp

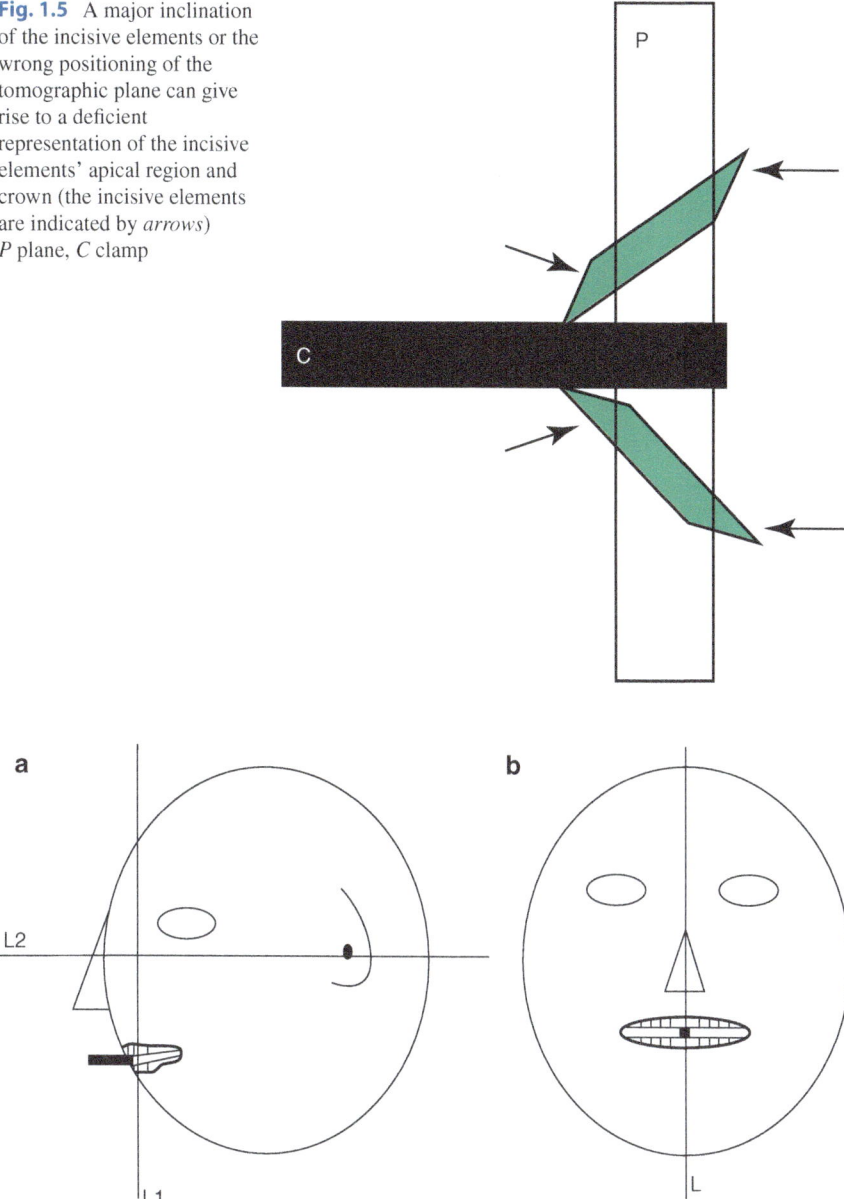

Fig. 1.6 (**a**) The lateral positioning is achieved by two luminous reference lines. *L1* corresponds to the tomographic plane, referring to the frontal group elements. *L2* represents the horizontal plane which must be aligned with the Frankfurt plane. (**b**) Positioning on the sagittal plane implies the use of a luminous reference line which divides the patient's face in two symmetrical halves. *L* luminous reference line

Fig. 1.7 Schematic diagram which describes the position of the 'water skier'. The body anteropulsion and the head retropulsion determine the withdrawal of the cervical spine

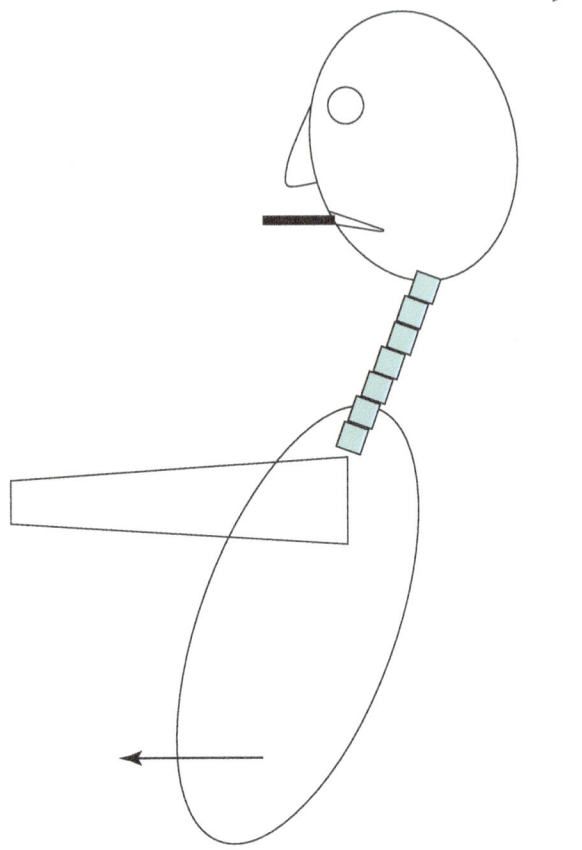

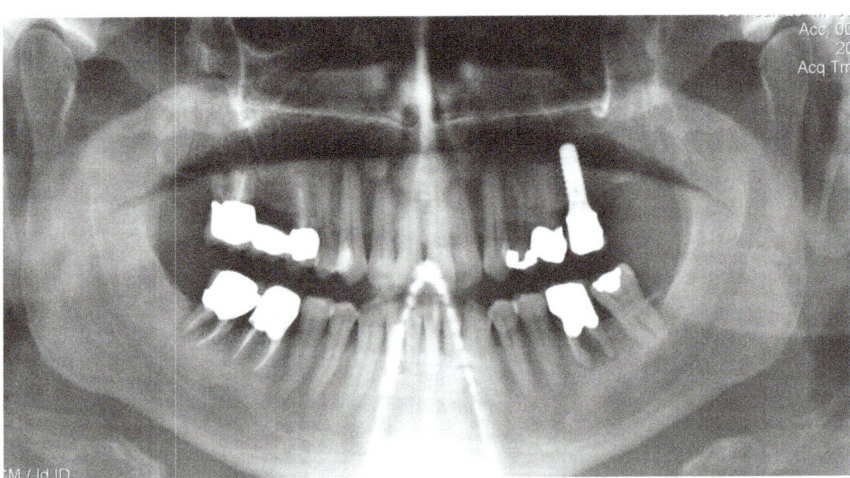

Fig. 1.8 Necklace artefact

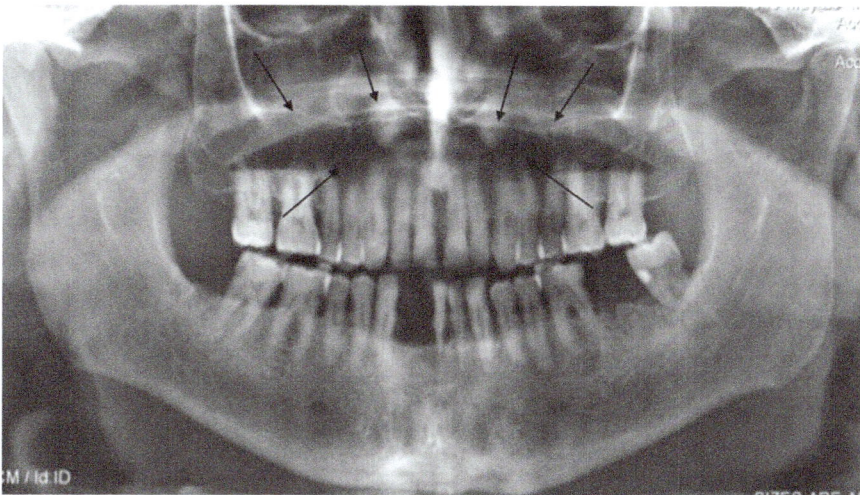

Fig. 1.9 Artefact caused by the missing apposition of the tongue. The radiolucency area (indicated by *arrows*) interferes with the reading of the superior arcade's apices

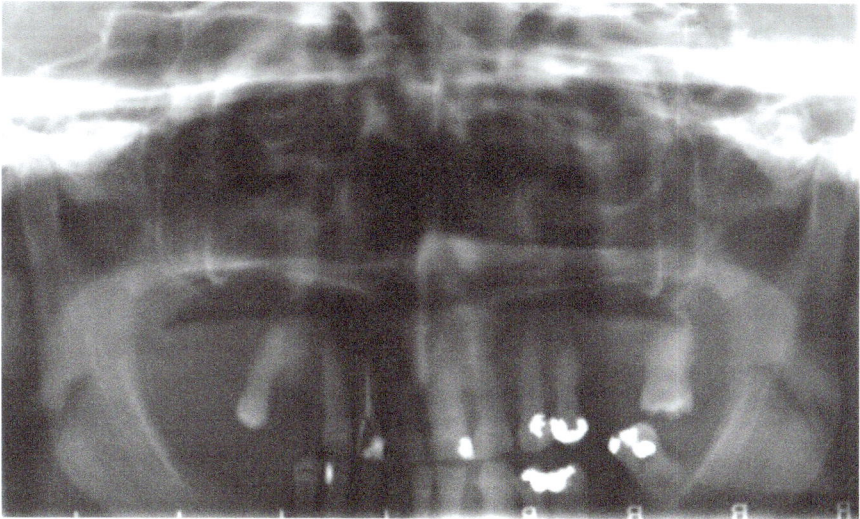

Fig. 1.10 Wrong positioning of the cassette

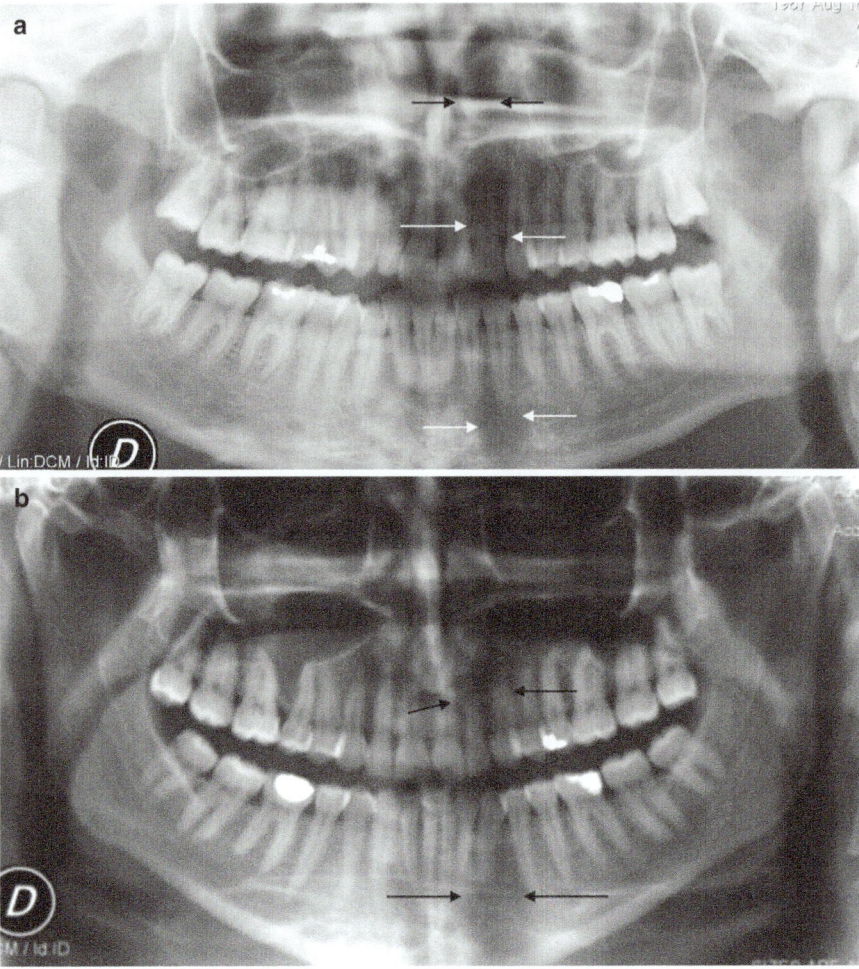

Fig. 1.11 (**a, b**) Overexposure bands (indicated by *arrows*) related to the slowing down of the tube detection system

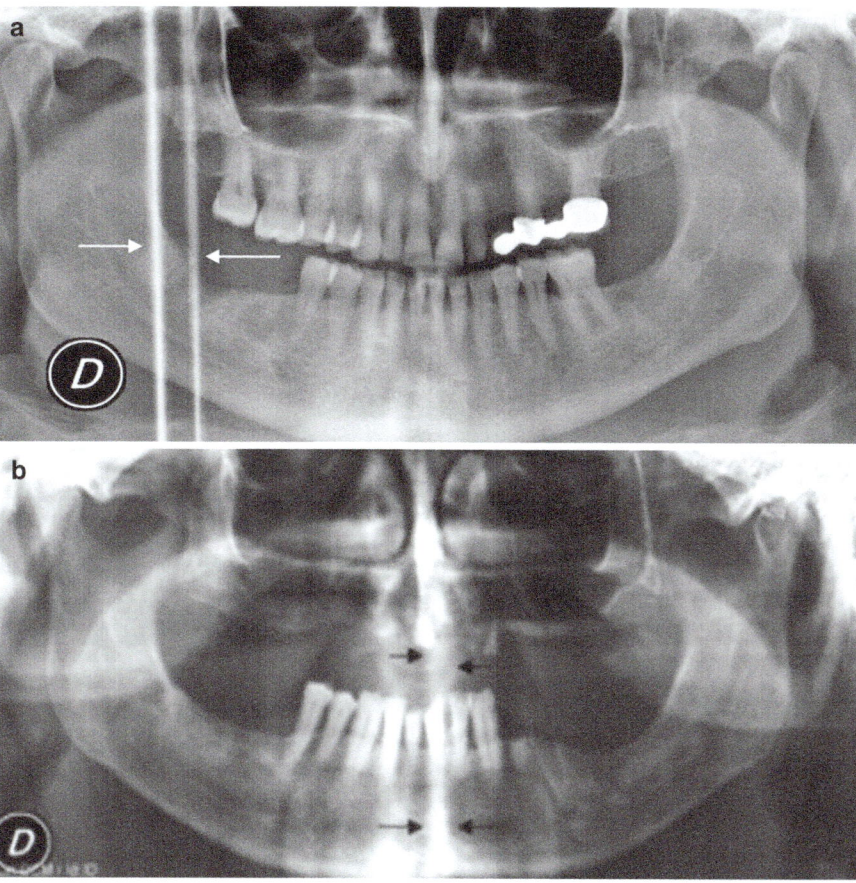

Fig. 1.12 (**a**) Underexposure double band (indicated by *arrows*) due to the momentaneous acceleration of the tube detection system or to the missing photon emission. (**b**) A similar artefact, projecting itself along the midline (indicated by *arrows*), hinders the reading of the inferior lateral left incisive tooth

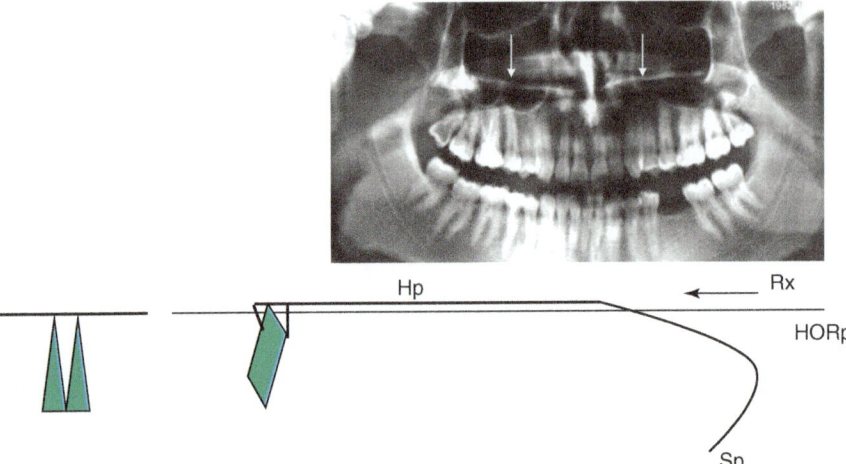

Fig. 1.13 Schematic diagram which illustrates the correct representation of the hard palate, aligned with the horizontal plane and caught by the radiant beam. It is shown as a thin radiopaque streak (indicated by *arrows*) which does not interfere with the visibility of the teeth apices. *Hp* hard palate, *Rx* radiant beam, *HORp* horizontal plane, *Sp* soft palate

Fig. 1.14 Schematic representation which illustrates the positive wrong inclination of the hard palate with respect to the horizontal plane. The apices of the incisive teeth come out from the tomographic plane. *HORp* horizontal plane, *P* plane, *Hp* hard palate, *Sp* soft palate

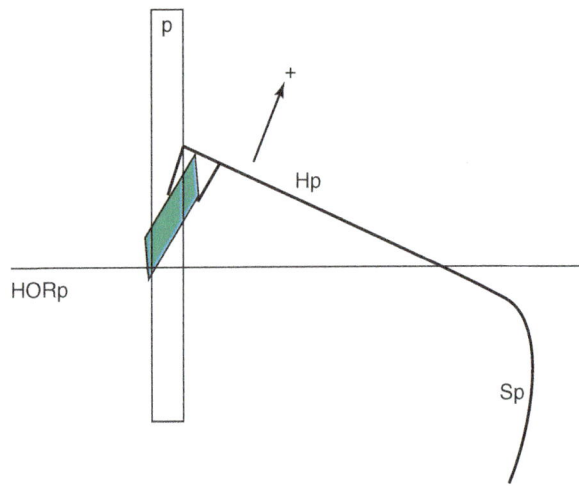

Fig 1.15 Schematic diagram which illustrates the negative wrong inclination of the hard palate with respect to the horizontal plane. The crown of the incisive teeth comes out from the tomographic plane, downwardly orienting itself. *HORp* horizontal plane, *P* plane, *Hp* hard palate, *Sp* soft palate

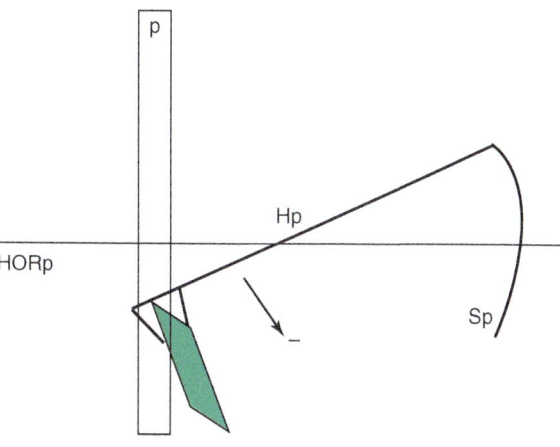

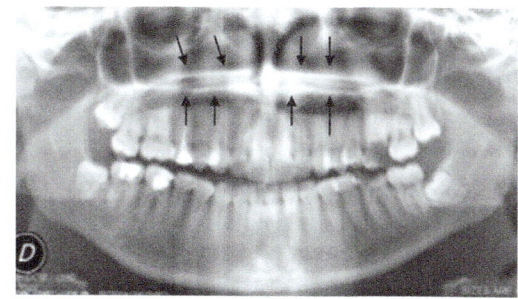

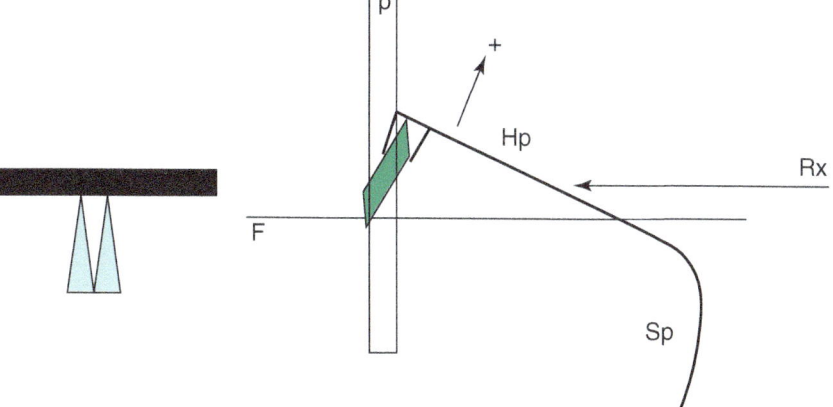

Fig. 1.16 Positive wrong inclination of the hard palate. The latter is represented by a radiopaque band which can interfere with the visibility of the teeth apices. The soft palate attempts to approach the detection plane. *F* Frankfurt plane, *P* plane, *Hp* hard palate, *Rx* radiant beam, *Sp* soft palate

Fig. 1.17 Transport of the soft palate (indicated by *long arrows*). Hyoid bone transport (indicated by *short arrow*) which interferes with the evaluation of the apices of the 37

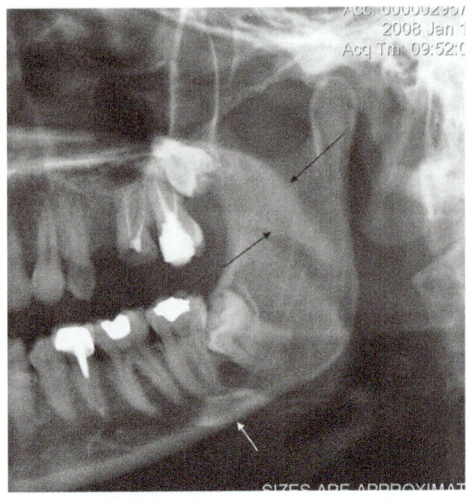

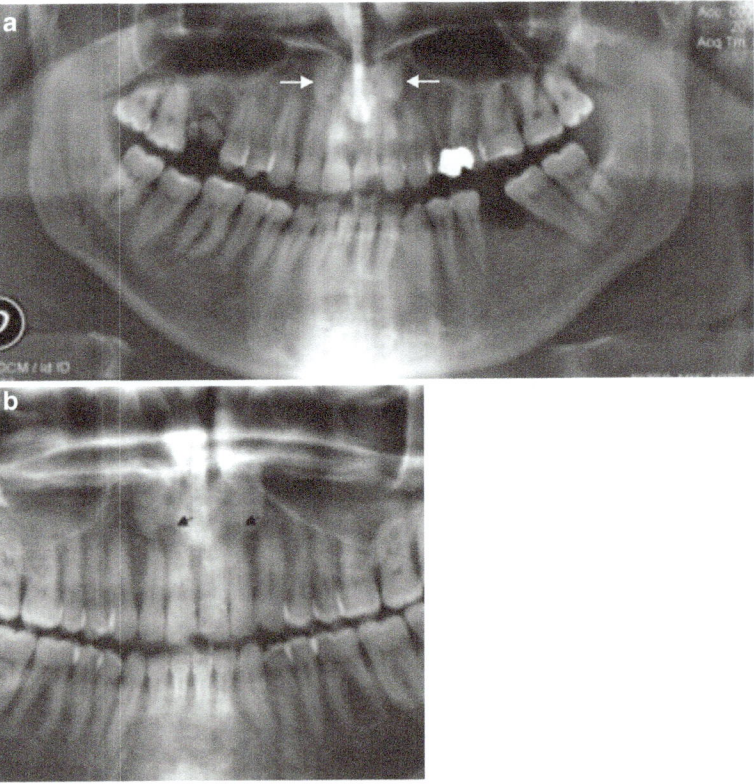

Fig. 1.18 (**a**) Artefact due to the nasal pyramid image of transport (indicated by *arrows*) which interferes with the analysis of the superior incisive teeth. (**b**) A similar artefact in which the radio-lucency of the nostrils (indicated by *arrows*) simulates the presence of periapical bone rarefaction's areas

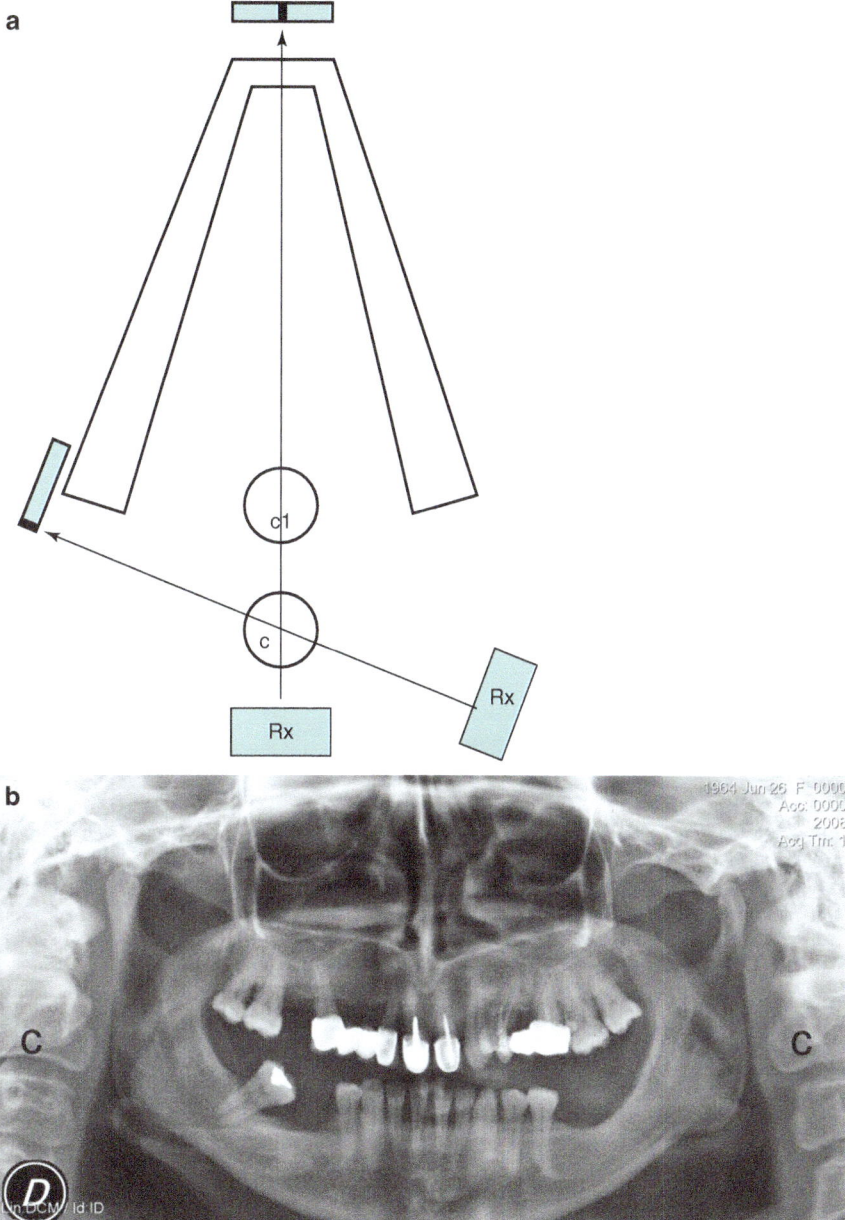

Fig 1.19 (**a**) Schematic diagram which shows the correct position of the cervical spine in relation to the tube detection system (the opacity of the cervical spine does not interfere with the image formation of the jawbone, projecting itself beyond it). Position $c1$ of the cervical spine is wrong as it is too far forwards. (**b**) Correct radiologic image in which the cervical spine projects itself out of the jawbone. *C* cervical spine, *Rx* radiant beam

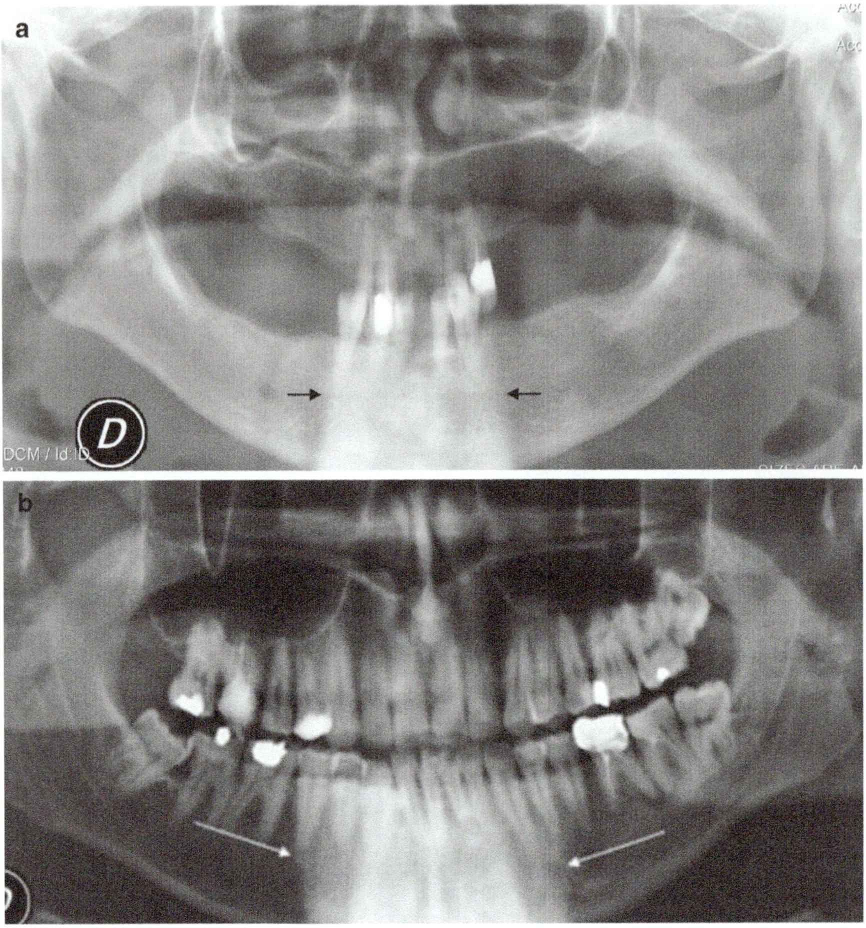

a

b

Fig. 1.20 (**a, b**) Artefact bands created by the cervical spine (indicated by *arrows*)

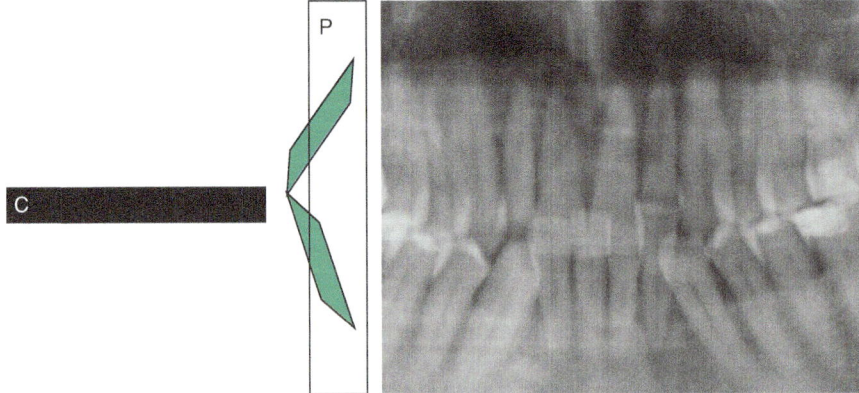

Fig. 1.21 Acquisition without clamp with occlusal juxtaposition of the incisive teeth can sometimes improve the visibility of the teeth apices, replacing them inside the tomographic plane. *C* clamp, *P* plane

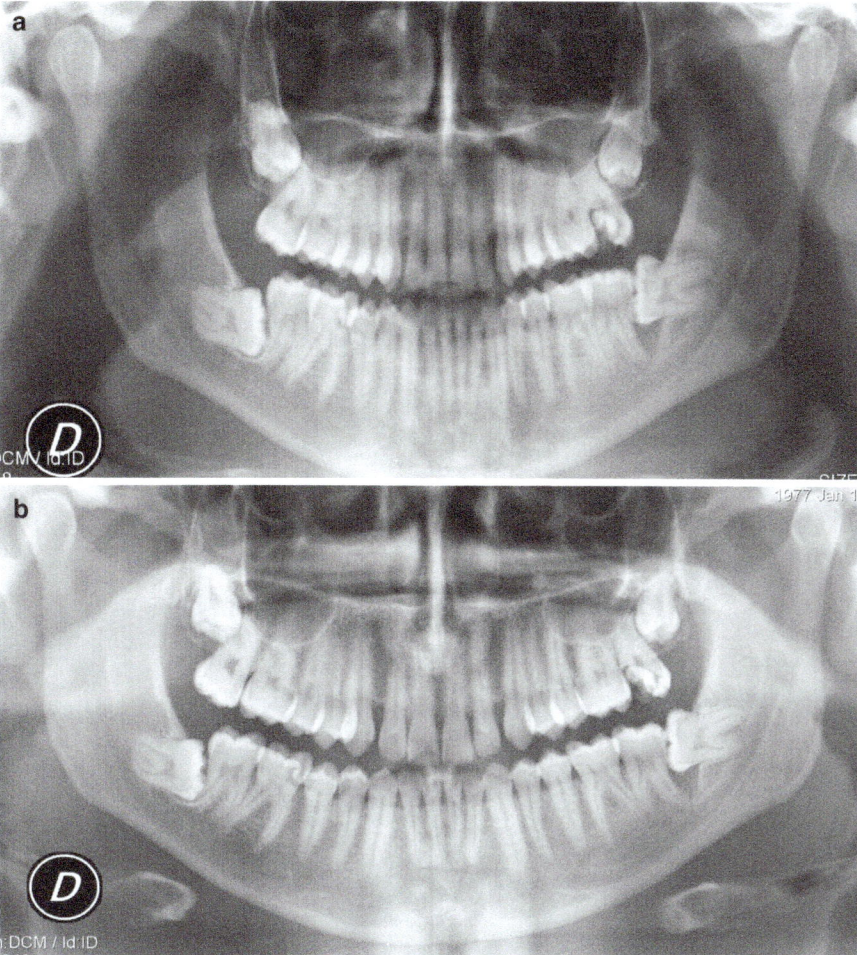

Fig. 1.22 (**a**) Head positioning too close to the detection plane. The dental arches turn out to be smaller with a consequent crowding of the dental elements. (**b**) A similar condition with correct positioning

Fig. 1.23 Wrong head positioning in relation to
the luminous reference line. One-half of the head will
be closer to the detection plane than the other one.
L luminous reference line

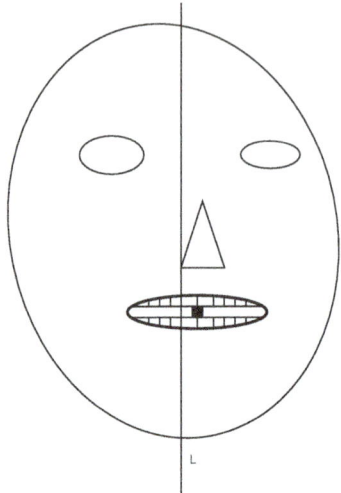

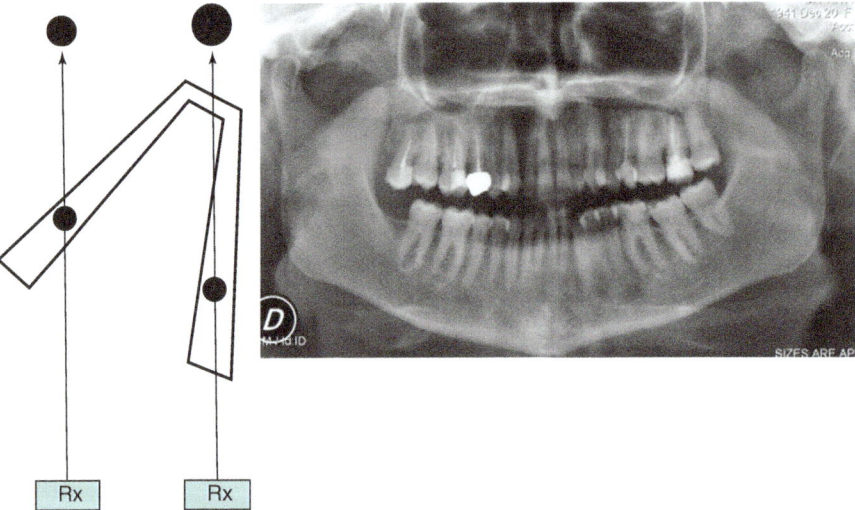

Fig. 1.24 Graphic representation of the positioning errors' effects of the head rotation, in relation
to the sagittal plane. In the radiogram the elements on the left turn out to be enlarged, as they are
farther from the detection plane. *Rx* radiant beam

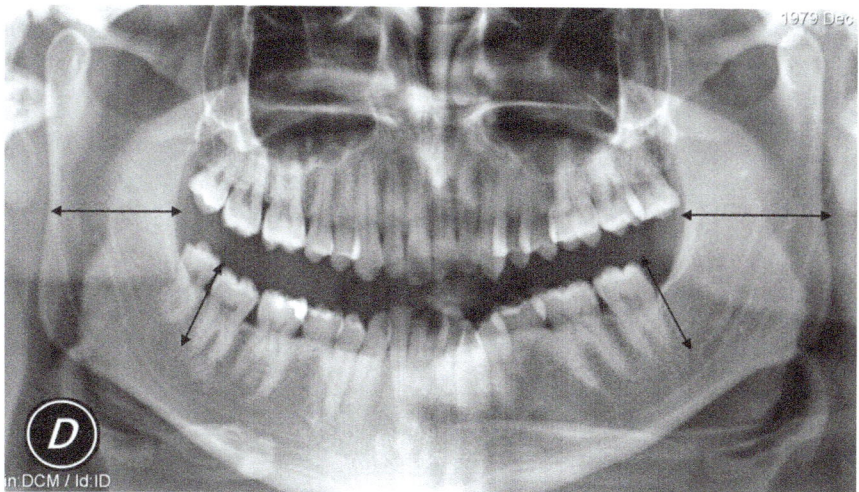

Fig. 1.25 Artefact due to asymmetrical enlargement. Horizontal enlargement is more evident in the mandibular branches (indicated by *arrows*). Longitudinal enlargement is more evident in the teeth (indicated by *arrows*)

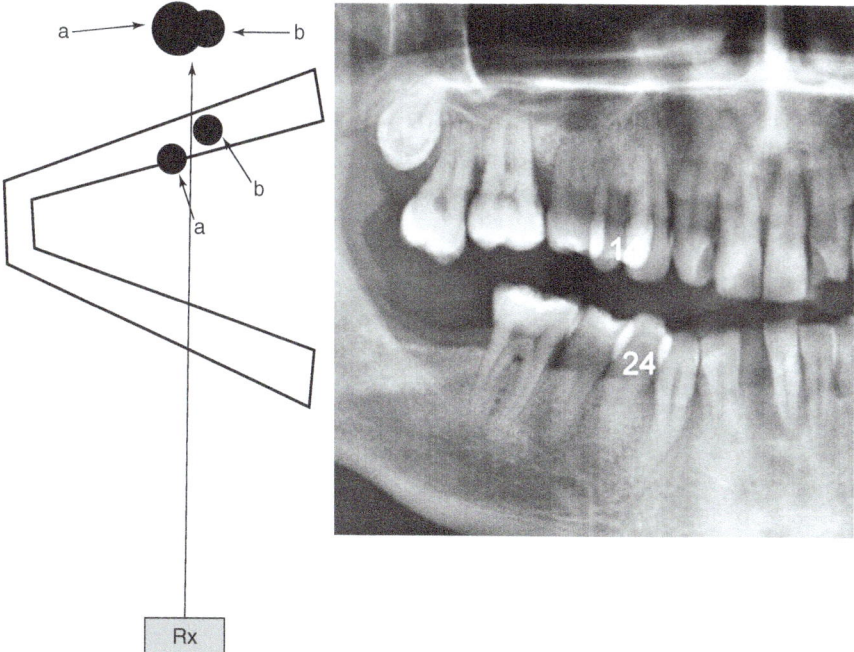

Fig. 1.26 Artefact due to interproximal superimposition. The scheme shows the element enlargement in the lingual seat (*a*) as it is farther from the detection plane than the element in normal position (*b*). The radiographic result is the interproximal superimposition of the elements 1.4 e 2.4 which are enlarged compared to the adjacent teeth. The interdental space is not visible. *Rx* radiant beam

Suggested Reading

Benson BW, Liang H, Flint DJ (2011) Panoramic radiography: digital technology fosters efficiency. Compend Contin Educ Dent 32(Spec No 4):6–8

Cederberg R (2012) Intraoral digital radiography: elements of effective imaging. Compend Contin Educ Dent 33(9):656–658, 662, 664

European Commission (2004) European guidelines on radiation protection in dental radiology. The safe use radiographs in dental practice, chapters 3, 4, 7. Office for official publications of the European Communities, Luxemburg

Gher ME, Richardson AC (1996) The accuracy of dental radiographic techniques used for evaluation of implant fixture placement. Int J Periodontics Restorative Dent 15(3):268–283

Kassebaum DK, Stoller NH, Goshorn BI (1992) Radiographic techniques for presurgical assessment of dental implant sites. Gen Dent 40(6):502–505, 509–510

Kraut RA (1993) Effective uses radiographs for implant placements: panographs, cephalographs, CT scans. Dent Implantol Update 4(4):29–33

Ladeira DB, Cruz AD, Almeida SM, Bóscolo FN (2012) Influence of the intergonial distance on image distortion in panoramic radiographs. Dentomaxillofac Radiol 41(5):417–421. Epub 2012 Jan 26

Lecomber AR, Yoneyama Y, Lovelock DJ, Hosoi T, Adams AM (2001) Comparison of patient dose from imaging protocols for dental implant planning using conventional radiography and computed tomography. Dentomaxillofac Radiol 30(5):255–259

Peretz B, Gotler M, Kaffe I (2012) Common errors in digital panoramic radiographs of patients with mixed dentition and patients with permanent dentition. Int J Dent 2012:584138. Epub 2012 Feb 8

Pfeiffer P, Bewersdorf S, Schmage P (2012) The effect of changes in head position on enlargement of structures during panoramic radiography. Int J Oral Maxillofac Implants 27(1):55–63

Pharoah MJ (1993) Imaging techniques and their clinical significance. Int J Prosthodont 6(2):176–179

Rout J, Brown J (2012) Ionizing radiation regulations and the dental practitioner: 1. The nature of ionizing radiation and its use in dentistry. Dent Update 39(3):191–192, 195–198, 201–203

Rout J, Brown J (2013) Object position and image magnification in dental panoramic radiography: a theoretical analysis. Dentomaxillofac Radiol 42:29951683

Normal Anatomy

2

In OPT, the evaluation of the masticatory normal anatomy is different for subjects of paediatric age and adults.

Indeed, subjects of paediatric age present a radiographic appearance which can be defined as '**mixed dentition**', in which **deciduous dental elements and permanent dental elements** coexist all together.

Therefore, in paediatric age, considerations of anatomic order and OPT possibilities are completely different from the ones applicable in the study of an adult subject.

We will firstly take into analysis the adult anatomy, with a completed dental development.

In the adult, the study of normal anatomy firstly is based on the definition of some general concepts, then subsequently a focused analysis on the following structures:

- **General anatomy of the tooth**
- **Anatomy of the support apparatus**
- **Anatomy of the mandible and the mandibular canal**
- **Anatomy of the surrounding structures** (paranasal sinuses, hard palate, nasal cavities, etc.)

Concepts of General Anatomy

The radiographic anatomy of the tooth in the adult, achievable through OPT, does not present the same detail refinement of the radiographic anatomy evaluated through endoral radiograms. This is due to the technical peculiarity of the methodology which favours a global vision rather than a detailed evaluation.

However, even if facing this limitation, dental images achieved through OPT are sufficient to fully express the macroscopical characteristics of the dental element, in the majority of the diagnostic needs.

I. Pandolfo, S. Mazziotti, *Orthopantomography*,
DOI 10.1007/978-88-470-5289-5_2, © Springer-Verlag Italia 2013

On the anatomical point of view, it is obviously necessary to take each of the dental typologies (incisors, canines, premolars and molars) into account separately.

In order to easily identify the different dental elements, a classical scheme is considered. It visualises the subdivision of the radiogram in four quadrants which are indicated with progressive numbers (1, 2, 3, 4), from right to left, from bottom up and clockwise.

Each number is associated to the relative dental element of each hemiarch. Number 1 indicates the median incisor, number 2 indicates the lateral incisor, number 3 indicates the canine, etc.

According to this method, for example, the third inferior right molar is indicated with number 4.8, the superior left canine is indicated with number 2.3, etc. (Fig. 2.1).

Such methodology, in addition to facilitating the detection of a specific dental element (in the OPT report), is also extremely useful for evaluating cases with alterations regarding the dental number, both in excess and, more rarely, in defect.

Descriptive and Radiographic Anatomy of the Dental Element

From the structural point of view, the tooth is an architectonical construction which comprises macroscopical and morphofunctional components. They have different purposes; therefore, they are constituted by different tissue types.

Indeed, the tooth is characterised by a visible component called **crown** and an intraosseous component called **root** (Fig. 2.2).

The dental crown represents the different functions of the tooth (shredding, stripping, section) through different morphologies (Fig. 2.3a, b).

The root is involved in the support apparatus and in the anchorage of the tooth to the jawbone.

The root end of the tooth is called **tooth apex** and it is characterised by a very thin hole which gives rise to the vascular-nervous axis.

The dental element, on its whole complex, is constituted by **dentin** which is an organic substance of mesodermic origin. It is covered by an external sheath called **enamel** (of ectodermal origin) in the crown and by the **cementum** (of mesodermic origin) in the root.

Therefore, the dentin is present both in the crown and in the root; it is composed of an organic component produced by the **odontoblasts** (about 30 %) and by a mineral component (about 70 %) which is composed of **hydroxyapatite crystals**.

Odontoblasts produce dentine in a dynamic manner both during the tooth's physiological development (**primary dentine**) and in pathological conditions (**secondary or reactive dentine**).

The enamel (produced by a cells called **ameloblasts**) covers the crown. Therefore, it turns out to be the seat of further mechanical stress; for this reason, it is composed of hydroxyapatite crystals for the 96 %.

Finally, the cementum is also composed of an organic matrix and a mineral component which determines the formation of the so-called mature cementum.

It covers the dentine at the level of the root axis line and is generated by **cementoblasts**. They are cellular elements placed in the tooth surface which are able to produce cementum for the whole life of the tooth.

Dental elements can be distinguished in monoradicular, biradicular and triradicular teeth.

As a general rule, even if subjected to numerous exceptions, it is possible to establish that incisors and canines of both arches turn out to be always monoradicular teeth. Moreover, all the premolars of the lower arch and the second premolars of the upper arch are monoradicular teeth, too.

Conversely, the first premolars of the upper arch generally have two roots (a vestibular one and a palatal one), while the first and the second molar of the lower arch (which are biradicular teeth, too) are characterised by a mesial and a distal root.

The first and the second molars of the upper arch always turn out to be triradicular teeth (having a mesial, a distal and a palatal root).

Finally, the third molars present a certain variability. They can be both monoradicular and, more rarely, biradicular teeth.

A transition area called **neck of tooth** or **cementoenamel junction** exists between the crown and the root. This is the area where the ameloblastic layer, represented by enamel, meets the root surface, which is constituted by the cement.

Inside the tooth, which presents a high radiopacity due to its structure, it is possible to recognise a radiolucency area which exist both in the crown and the root. Such area is, respectively, the expression of the **pulp chamber** and the **root canal** (Fig. 2.4).

The root canal is characterised by very thin horizontal and oblique collateral canals, called **lateral canals** (however, they are never radiographically visible).

Vascular-nervous elements exist both in the pulp chamber and in the root canal. Together with a connective support (of mesodermic origin) they constitute the **dental pulp**.

The dental pulp has three purposes: dentine formation (**dentinogenesis**) and both nutritive and sensorial functions.

To conclude this general analysis of the dental anatomy, it must be remembered that from a topographic point of view, each tooth is characterised by a face which is oriented towards the cheek, called **vestibular surface**, and another face which is oriented towards the tongue, called **lingual surface**.

Another face fulfils the mastication process and is particularly augmented in the molars. It is called the **occlusal surface** as it is influenced, in its morphology, by juxtaposition or **occlusal rapports** with the dental elements of the opposed arch.

Furthermore, two other faces exist. One face, directed towards the median line, is called **mesial surface** and another face, opposed to it, is called **distal surface**. They are interfaces between two dental elements, thereby called **interproximal surfaces** (Fig. 2.5).

As aforementioned, this distinction is also valid for the denomination of the root axis surfaces. Indeed, in a triradicular element, it is possible to distinguish the mesial root from the distal one, in addition to the third root, called palatal. The latter seems to be typically present at the level of the first and the second upper molars and it is not always demonstrable through OPT, for projective reasons.

Indeed, the **palatal root** develops itself in a different plane with respect to the other roots.

As it is placed farther from the detection plane, it will turn out to be radiographically less defined and rather enlarged (Fig. 2.6a, b).

It is obvious that the aforementioned expressions of topographic and semantic order are absolutely necessary in order to localise the morbid processes. Therefore, they are propaedeutical to a correct draft of the radiological report.

Descriptive and Radiological Anatomy of the Support Apparatus or Periodontium

The anatomical and functional structure is responsible for the stability of the dental elements, and in final analysis, of the whole masticatory apparatus. It is constituted by the following components: the **gingiva**, the **periodontal ligament (PDL)** and the **alveolar bone**, which in turn is constituted by the spongiosa and the cortical plate (**lamina dura**). According to some experts, the cementum is part of the alveolar bone, too (Fig. 2.7).

OPT allows a panoramic evaluation of the normal anatomy and, consequently, of the pathological alterations related only to some of the aforementioned components.

Indeed, it is well known that the evaluation of the gingival apparatus is exclusively of clinical pertinence and also a direct radiographic visualisation of the periodontal ligament is not possible. As a consequence, the state of the periodontal ligament can be indirectly evaluated according to the extent of the periodontal space which, in a normal subject, turns out to be radiographically invisible or scarcely detectable.

Therefore, the radiographic representation of the periodontal apparatus is referred only to the analysis of the alveolar bone, which is constituted by **interdental and intraradicular cuspids**, with their relative components (spongiosa and lamina dura). Moreover, it is also referred to the evaluation of the periodontal space extent and to the state of the dental roots (Fig. 2.8).

The periodontal space is a thin radiolucent line which hosts the namesake ligament, constituted by collagen fibres produced by **fibroblasts**. Fibroblasts originate from the embryonic cellular elements which are contained in the dental sac.

The elements of the aforementioned ligament-fibrous apparatus (**Sharpey's fibres**) are hooked up to the cementum and to the cortical plate of the bundle bone at the level of the alveolar face.

Descriptive and Radiographic Anatomy of the Mandible and the Mandibular Canal

The anatomy of the mandible, evaluable through OPT, can be synthetically described as follows.

Analogous with the classic anatomical literature, it is possible to distinguish the **ascending branch** or **mandibular ramus**. Anteriorly, it gives rise to the **coronoid apophysis** (insertion area of the **temporal muscle**) and posteriorly to the **intercondylar region** and the **mandibular condyle**, in which the articular relationships with the **glenoid cavity** are well rendered.

Distally, the ascending branch continues with the interposition of the **mandibular angle** (**angular region**), with the **mandibular body** or **horizontal branch**. At the level of the median line, there is the **symphysis menti** region.

In the angular region is present a superior surface with triangular morphology, covered by the gingiva. This angular region is set behind the last molar and is called **retromolar trigone**. It is the anatomical area of major importance for oncological implications.

Moreover, the mandibular angle, in the inferior lateral side, is characterised by irregular salience and roughness. It represents the insertion area of the **masseter muscle** (Fig. 2.9a, b).

In its complex, the mandible is constituted by a bundle of cortical bone tissue which is characterised by a major thickness in the lower part and by the sponge tissue which represents the medullary bone.

The sponge tissue presents a different architecture and a different grade of opacity, depending on the age, the nutritional state and the general skeletal trophism of the patients.

At the level of the horizontal branch and of the angular region, it is possible, in many subjects, to detect a major opacity band which indicates the **ridge (of insertion) of the mylohyoid muscle**. The band is situated at the level of the vestibular surface which is better evident in edentulous subjects for the hypotrophy of the surrounding bone (Fig. 2.10).

More cranially, in the ascending branch, it is possible to demonstrate the entry foramen of the **mandibular canal** and a little bone salience adjacent to it, called **Spix spine**. The Spix spine is the insertion of the **fibrous pterygomandibular raphe**, which in turn is never demonstrable through the OPT examination (Fig. 2.11).

Conversely, in almost all the patients, it is possible to radiographically demonstrate the mandibular canal into which the **inferior alveolar nerve** runs. The inferior alveolar nerve is the medial ramus of the **mandibular nerve**, which is the third branch of the **trigeminal nerve**.

As the mandibular canal is a bone channel delimitated by a thin cortical side, in OPT, it assumes the peculiar aspect of a canalicular structure. This structure has a low density and a diameter of 1.5–2 mm. Its proximal extremity is, in turn, characterised by a funnel morphology which is the entrance of the nerve (Fig. 2.12a, b).

As the mandibular canal runs into a spongeous bone tissue, its visibility in OPT is closely related to the opacity grade of the surrounding spongiosa.

In the subjects with a high level of osteopenia, which causes the absence of optimal contrast conditions, a scarce or absent visualisation of the mandibular canal can occur. In this case, the medical report cannot be considered pathological.

Conversely, in the presence of high bone density, the visibility of the channel can be better (Fig. 2.13a, b).

If radiological visibility is good, it is easy to visualise the curvilinear aspect of the canal in its horizontal portion, as well as the aforementioned funnel aspect of its proximal extremity. The anterior segment up to the opening of the **mental foramen** will also be visible. The mental foramen, most frequently, corresponds to the apex of the second premolar tooth (Fig. 2.14).

In regard to this, in the majority of cases, the missing visualisation of such foramen is due to projective reasons; therefore, it cannot be considered a pathological event.

A further consideration is represented by the possible variability of the mental foramen seat.

Indeed, if it is not perfectly matched with the typical position, it cannot be considered pathological but a normal anatomical variation.

As a matter of fact, the mental foramen can be located both in correspondence with the apex of the second premolar tooth and at a certain distance from it. More rarely, it can be placed at the apex of the first premolar tooth.

Errors related to such variability are infrequent and made only by inexpert observers who may wrongly interpret the mental foramen radiolucency as the periapical lesion of the second premolar tooth (Fig. 2.15a, b).

This can be easily avoided through comparison with the contralateral normal side. Obviously, the absolute normality of the dental element under exam must be evaluated.

As mentioned earlier, it is sometimes possible to provide evidence of the very thin **incisive canaliculus** as a characteristic of normal anatomy. It leads itself from the mental foramen towards the elements of the inferior incisive bundle (Fig. 2.16).

Moreover, the other **dental canaliculi** are rarely and occasionally visible in normal anatomy (Fig. 2.17).

An outstanding anatomical variant, to be considered in implantological planning, is represented by the **bend** that the **mandibular canal** accomplishes in its more distal portion, before its opening into the mental foramen.

In a few words, the canal, at such a level, can create a curve (also called **loop of the mandibular canal**). This is directed in front and towards the median line. It then folds back and returns to the mental foramen (Fig. 2.18).

It seems to be clear that, if this anatomical configuration is not indicated, it can negatively reverberate during an implantologic intervention in this region.

Indeed, it is known that the second inferior premolar is considered to be the external anatomical landmark, corresponding to the mental foramen, which identifies the distal limit of the alveolar nerve.

It is obvious that the presence of a marked **loop of the mandibular canal** places the nerve in a more mesial seat with respect to the second premolar tooth.

This configuration can determine the iatrogenic lesion of the nerve, as a consequence of surgical operations performed at such level.

The rare possibility of mandibular canal bifidity must always be remembered with regard to the anatomical variations. It is also considered to be an important anatomical variation in the programmes of implantologic planning (Fig. 2.19).

Finally, the duplicity of the mandibular canal represents a more significant and rare condition from the clinical point of view, as it is linked (demonstrated only in a few cases in literature) to the presence of neoformations of vascular origin (arterio-venous fistula). One of the two canals represents the course of the nerve; the other canal represents the path of the afferent vascular structures to the aforementioned lesions (Fig. 2.20).

Anatomical variants are often deprived of any pathological significance, but sometimes they are the cause of clinical sintomathology and/or of complications after tooth extraction.

Considering those variants, the mandibular canal and the third molar tooth can interface between them in numerous ways. Indeed, according to this variability, some risks can occur. These include the transference of pathological events from the dental element to the canal and iatrogenic damages related to tooth extraction.

It is obvious that the relevance of the security distance between the tooth and the canal involves minor risks (Fig. 2.21).

Conversely, a close adjacency between the dental element and the canal determines major risk conditions (Fig. 2.22a–c).

In regard to this, disappearance of one of the canal cortical, in adjacency to the tooth is an important semeiological finding.

Such disappearance could indicate the real contact between the two structures. Conversely, where the cortical is visible, even in correspondence with the tooth, it must be considered that the structures are not in contact but only superimposed projectively.

Briefly, such semeiological sign is an extension of the **silhouette sign**, very well known in general radiographic semeiotics (Fig. 2.23a, b).

Finally, the aforementioned iatrogenic risks become more relevant in case of anomalies of position and orientation of the third molar tooth.

In particular, the inclusion of the third molar tooth, increasing the proximity of the tooth to the canal, represents a significant risk condition, along with its frequency (Fig. 2.24a–c).

Furthermore, it has to be to be considered that CT can exhaustively define the real space relations between the tooth and the canal, thanks to its tridimensional approach. This is not possible using OPT as it is only able to define the aforementioned relations bidimensionally.

Anatomy of the Surrounding Structures

Therefore, the surrounding structures of the dental arches which are visible in OPT mainly include **maxillary sinuses**, **nasal cavities**, **hard palate**, **pterygoid apophysis**, **pterygopalatine fossae**, **temporomandibular joints** and **zygomatic arches** (Fig. 2.25a, b).

It is obvious that the analytical evaluation of the aforementioned structures (except the temporomandibular joints, whose analysis does not belong to the aims of the following text) is not the fundamental aim of OPT, as the imaging of such areas always pertain to other techniques of major efficiency such as CT and MR.

However, it is evident that the radiologist must be able to recognise such anatomical structures and their more common variants (Fig. 2.26); in addition, he must be able to detect any possible anomalies, indicating the most suitable imaging techniques.

From this viewpoint, some alterations of the skeletal components of the facial bones seem to be paradigmatic, such as those related to fibrous dysplasia, osteolytic lesions, palatoschisis and osteomatous formations (Figs. 2.27, 2.28, and 2.29).

The content of the maxillary sinuses can also be the seat of pathological events which generically occur as endoluminal opacity. Most of the times they are considered innocuous **retentive pseudocysts**, but they can be in differential diagnosis both with other pathological events (polyposis, neoplasia) and with particular anatomical variations (Fig. 2.30a, b).

Finally, the possibility of anomalies of odontogenic origin must not be ignored. These anomalies are characterised by an endosinusal development and will be discussed subsequently in the text.

Radiographic Anatomy in Paediatric Age

As previously explained, the aspect of the masticatory apparatus in paediatric age turns out to be very different to that of the adult.

As a consequence, both age groups have entirely distinct radiographic cases and descriptive terminology.

However, for both age groups, the same scheme is used for the function of identifying and enumerating the dental elements.

The study sector can be subdivided into four quadrants: considering as number 5 the superior right hemiarch, number 6 the superior left hemiarch, number 7 the inferior left hemiarch and number 8 the inferior right hemiarch.

As the deciduous dental elements are 5 for each hemiarch, they are detected (similarly to the adults) with the following numbers: 5.1 refers to the superior median right incisor, 6.1 refers to its corresponding left tooth and so on (see Fig. 2.31).

This calculation must obviously consider the fact that the development of molar teeth does not precede the appearance of deciduous dental elements.

Also from the morphological point of view, there is a substantial difference between the deciduous dental elements and the permanent ones. The deciduous dental elements present minor dimensions; they have a somewhat squat aspect and some distinct morphological connotations: for example, a characteristic of the deciduous premolar teeth is a biradiculated aspect.

In addition, the deciduous elements, under the push of the underlying permanent elements, present a variable grade of radicular reabsorption, which is called **rhizolysis** or **physiological apicolysis** (it has to be distinguished from the **pathological**

rhizolysis which can appear in the adult in presence of periapical-flogistic lesions) (Fig. 2.32).

Also the permanent dental elements, while still in the phase of dehiscence, present significant morphological and dimensional differences, with respect to the same elements already developed.

They present a more or less incomplete development of the radicular axes, which appear to be short or not present, when compared to their fully developed state. For the same reason, the apical foramen is very wide (Fig. 2.33).

In order to better understand the main morphological characteristics of the permanent tooth still in phase of dehiscence, some preliminary remarks are essential in regard to the embryogenetic development.

The dental germ (both the deciduous and permanent one) originates from an introflexion of the dental ridge. It turns out to be entirely surrounded by a thin membrane called **dental sac** (or **alveolar sac**). Its primary function is protection.

In its interior, the dental germ appears further lined by a membrane composed of an internal layer attached to the crown germ. This is the seat of ameloblasts (cells of ectodermic origin, responsible for the formation of the enamel). The dental germ is also covered by an external layer in contact with the dental sac.

Between the aforementioned membranes, there is a certain amount of mesenchymal tissue which basically has a trophic function, called **stellate reticulum**.

The aforementioned anatomical-functional structure takes the name of **organ of the enamel** and it is responsible for the whole tooth development. In particular it is responsible for the construction of the normal enamel shell of the crown dentine.

Even if it varies in relation to the evolutionary state, it is nearly always radiographically detectable (Fig. 2.34).

The organ of the enamel represents a critical structure. This is due to the cystic degeneration of the mesenchymal component, which constitutes the stellate reticulum, and is the basis for odontogenic follicular cyst formation.

Image Gallery

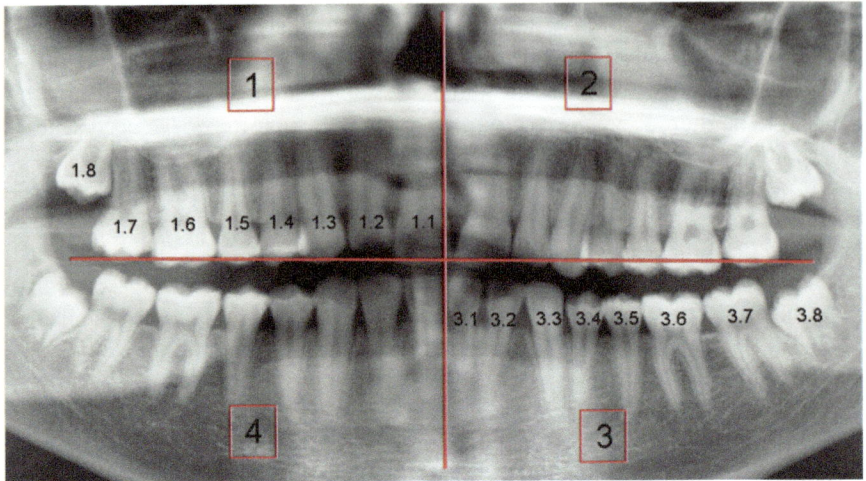

Fig. 2.1 Scheme showing the topographic detection of the dental elements

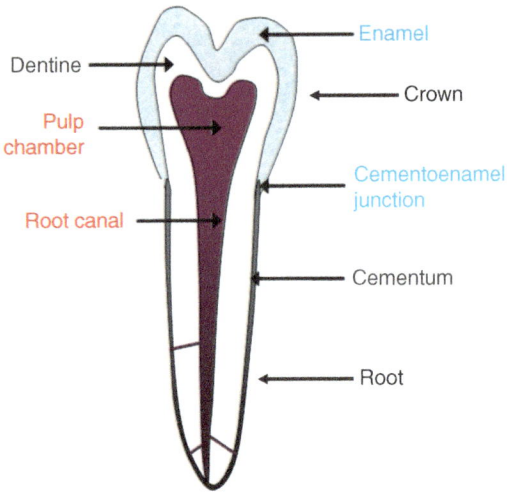

Fig. 2.2 Schematic diagram which illustrates the different morphological and structural components of the tooth

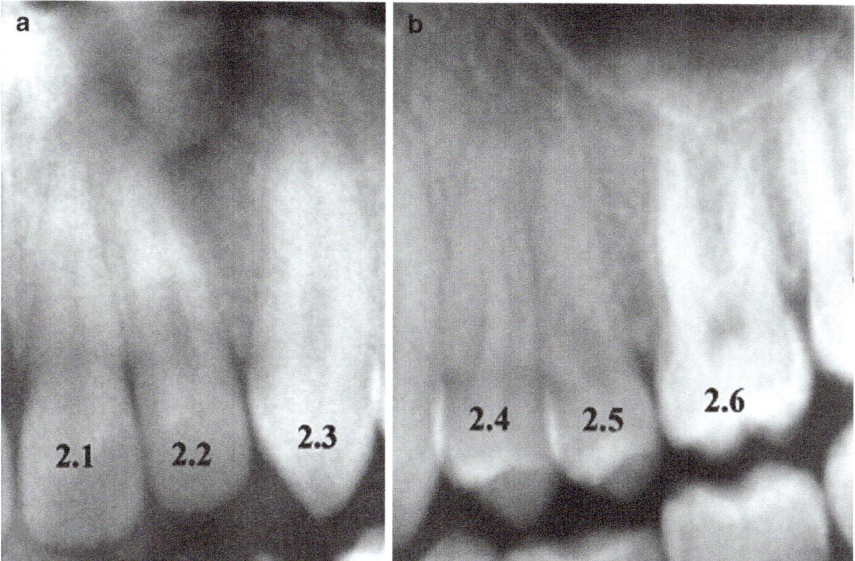

Fig. 2.3 (**a**) Crown morphology of the median and lateral incisors and of the left canine (2.1, 2.2 e 2.3) aiming at stripping. (**b**) Crown morphology of the premolars 2.4 and 2.5 and of the first left molar (2.6) aiming at shredding

Fig. 2.4 The *long red arrow* indicates the enamel characterised by maximum opacity. The *short red arrow* indicates the cementoenamel junction. The *long yellow arrow* indicates the pulp chamber. The *short yellow arrows* indicate the radicular canals

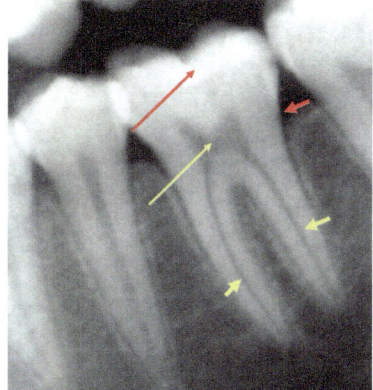

Fig. 2.5 *1* Vestibular surface. *2* Lingual (or palatal) surface. *3* Occlusal surface. *4* Distal surface. *5* Mesial surface

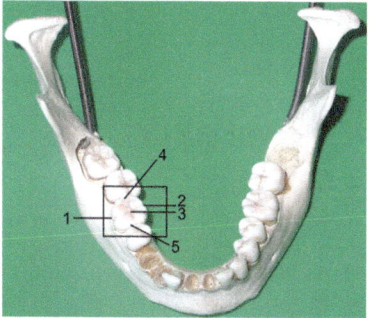

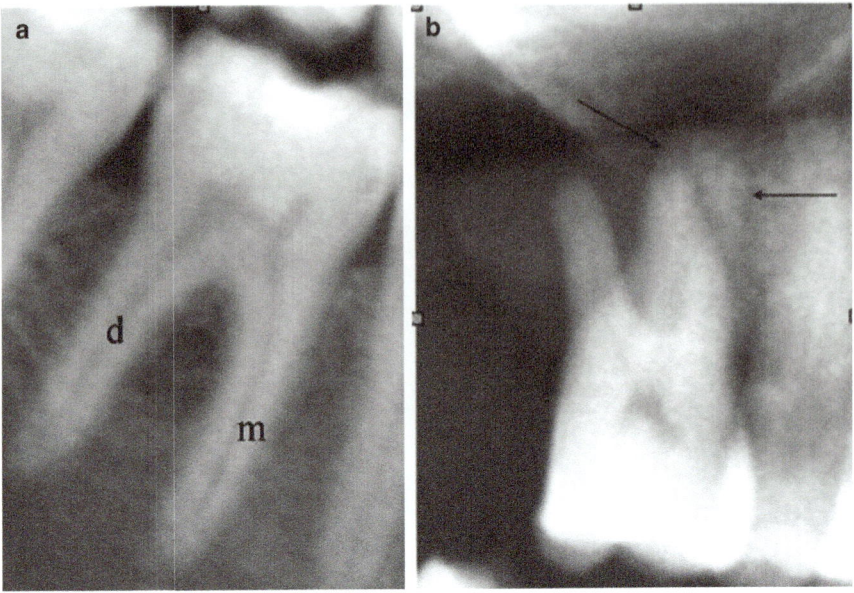

Fig. 2.6 (**a**) The image shows the biradicular tooth; letter 'd' indicates the distal root; letter 'm' indicates the mesial root. (**b**) The image shows the triradicular tooth. The palatal root (indicated by *arrows*) seems to be enlarged with blurred outlines

Fig. 2.7 Schematic diagram which represents the periodontium

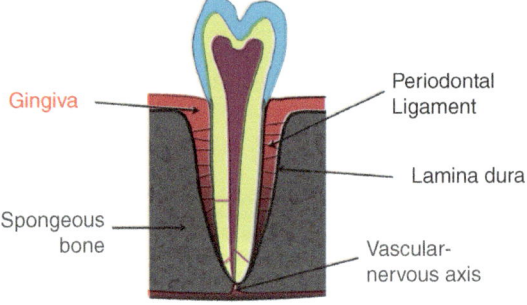

Fig. 2.8 Radiographic representation of the periodontal apparatus. The *arrowhead* indicates the periodontal space; the *yellow arrow* indicates the lamina dura; the *green star* indicates the spongiosa of the interadicular cuspid; the *asterisk* indicates the spongiosa of the interdental cuspid

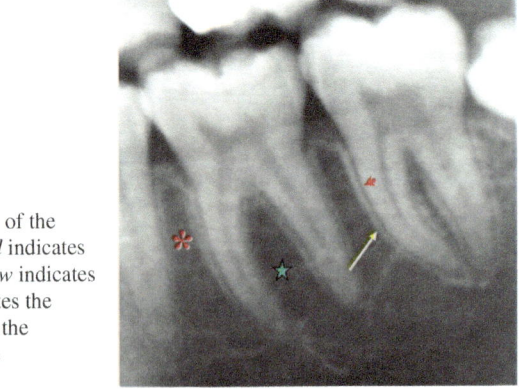

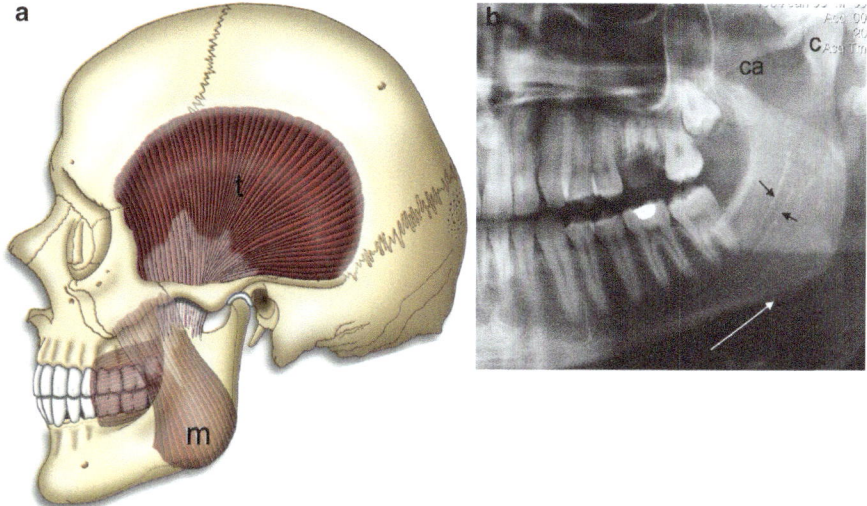

Fig. 2.9 (**a**) Anatomical diagram which shows the insertion of the masseter muscle (*m*) into the angular region of the mandible. The temporal muscle (*t*) inserts itself into the coronoid apophysis. (**b**) Radiogram which shows the main elements of the mandible: Letter 'c' stands for condyle; letters 'ca' stands for coronoid apophysis; the *short arrows* indicate the mandibular canal; the *long arrow* indicates the cortical roughness which is due to the insertion of the masseter muscle

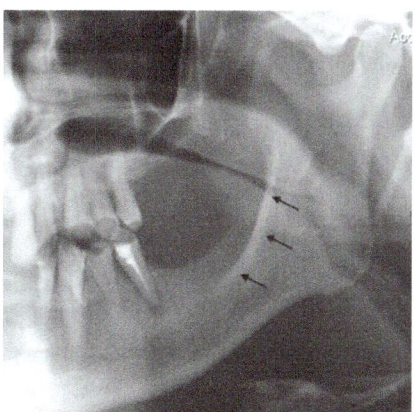

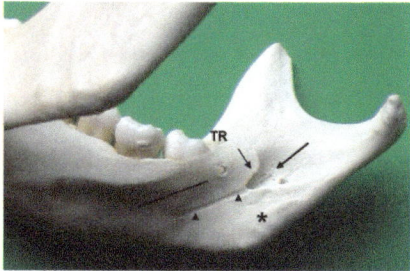

Fig. 2.10 The mylohyoid muscle ridge (indicated by *arrows*) is clearly visible

Fig. 2.11 Anatomical photo which shows the entry foramen of the mandibular canal (indicated by *long arrow*). The *short arrow* indicates the Spix spine. The *arrow heads* indicate the sulcus of the mylohyoid nerve. The *asterisk* indicates the insertion area of the internal pterygoid muscle. *TR* retromolar trigone. The black line indicates the mylohyoid bony ridge

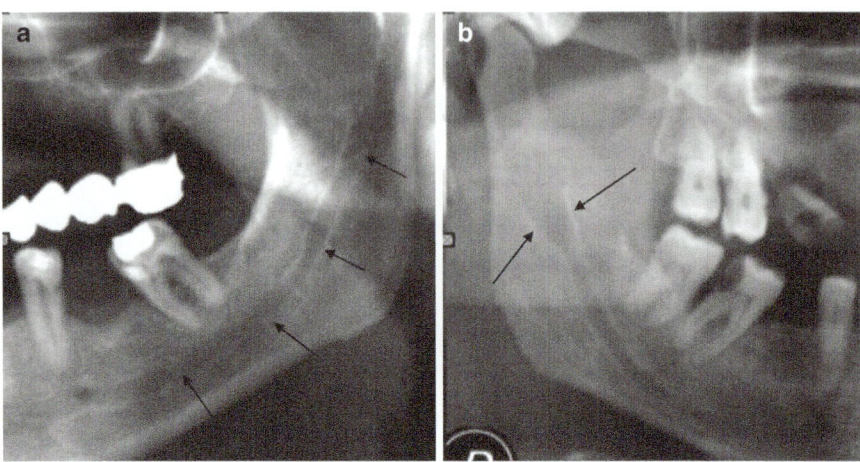

Fig. 2.12 (**a**) Good visibility of the mandibular canal (indicated by *short arrows*). (**b**) Funnel aspect of the mandibular canal in its proximal extremity (indicated by *long arrows*)

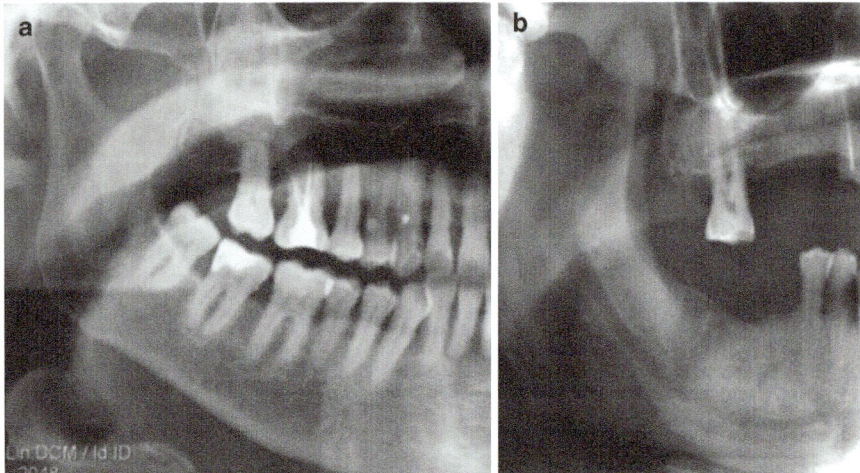

Fig. 2.13 (**a**) Scarce visibility of the mandibular canal in (a) patient with hypotrophy of the spongiosa. (**b**) Optimal visibility of the mandibular canal due to the sclerosis of the surrounding spongiosa

Fig. 2.14 Mental foramen (indicated by *arrow*) in its typical collocation which is in proximity to the apex of the second premolar (3.5)

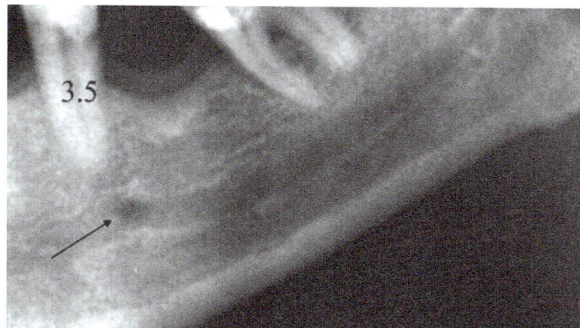

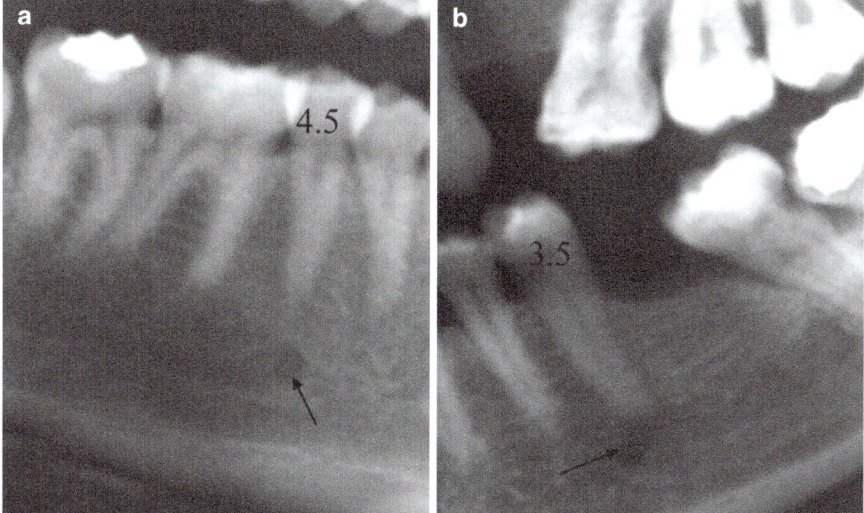

Fig. 2.15 (**a, b**) Variability of the mental foramen seat (indicated by *arrows*). In (a) the mental foramen is at a certain distance from the apex of the second inferior right premolar (4.5). In (b) the foramen is adjacent to the second inferior left premolar (3.5) and it must not be interpreted as a periapical area of bone resorption

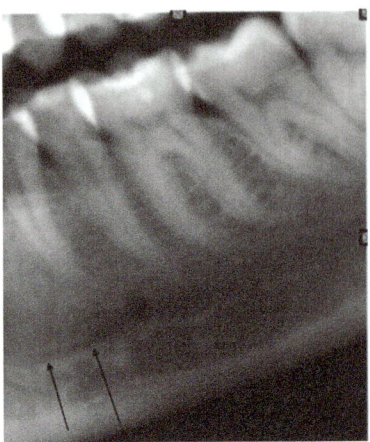

Fig. 2.16 It is possible to provide evidence of the incisive canaliculus (indicated by *arrows*) which leads itself from the mental foramen towards the inferior central elements

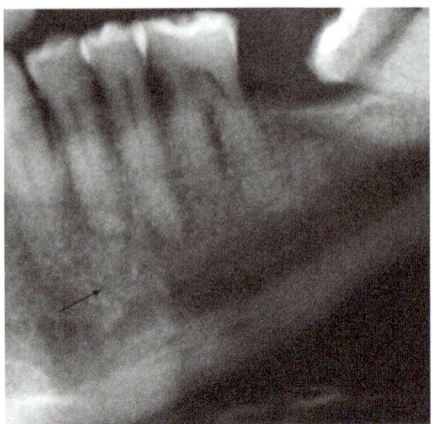

Fig. 2.17 Occasional visibility of a dental canaliculus (represented by *arrow*) in normal anatomy

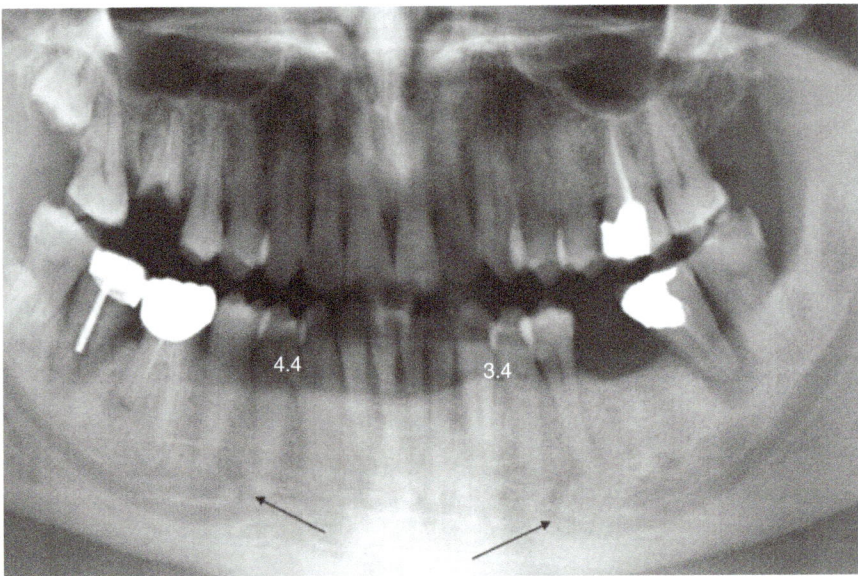

Fig. 2.18 Bend of the mandibular canal (indicated by *arrows*). This configuration determines the mandibular canal's approach to the region corresponding to the first premolar on each side (3.4 e 4.4)

Fig. 2.19 Bifidity of the right mandibular canal (indicated by *short arrow*) following a fistulous path towards the apex (indicated by *long arrow*) of the mesial root of the 4.6

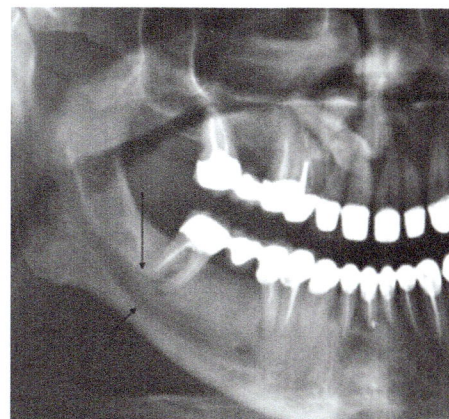

Fig. 2.20 Real duplicity of the mandibular canal (indicated by *arrows*). The superior canal gives way to the path of vascular structures and widens into a lacunar image (*F*), which is the expression of the arteriovenous fistula

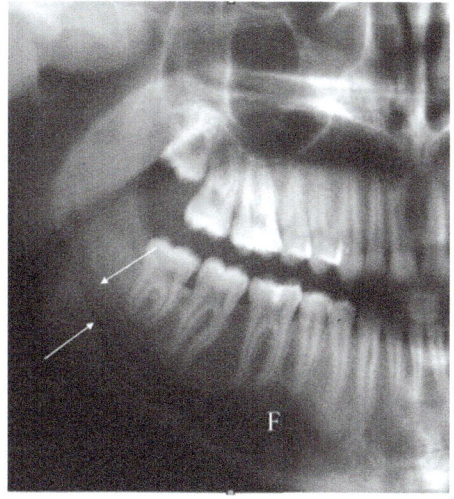

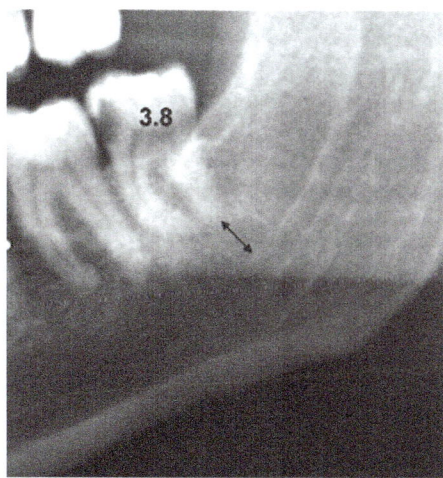

Fig. 2.21 Wide security distance between the apex of the 3.8 and the mandibular canal double side *arrow*

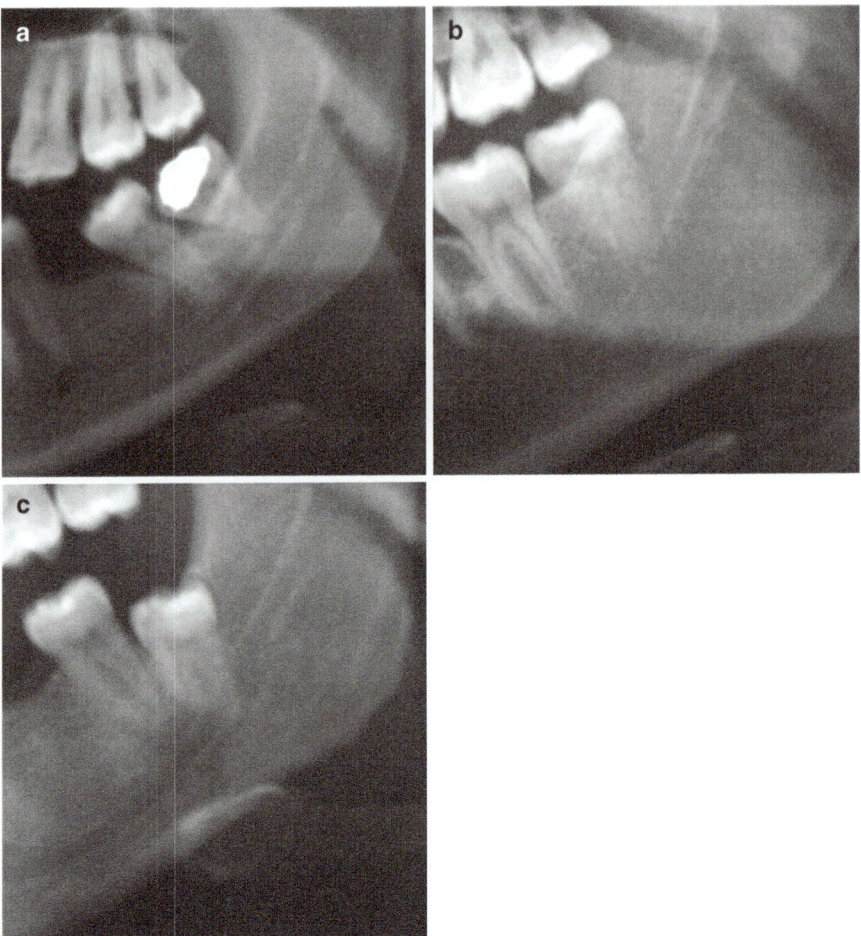

Fig. 2.22 (**a–c**) Different 'critical' situations of the rapports between the third molar (3.8) and the mandibular canal

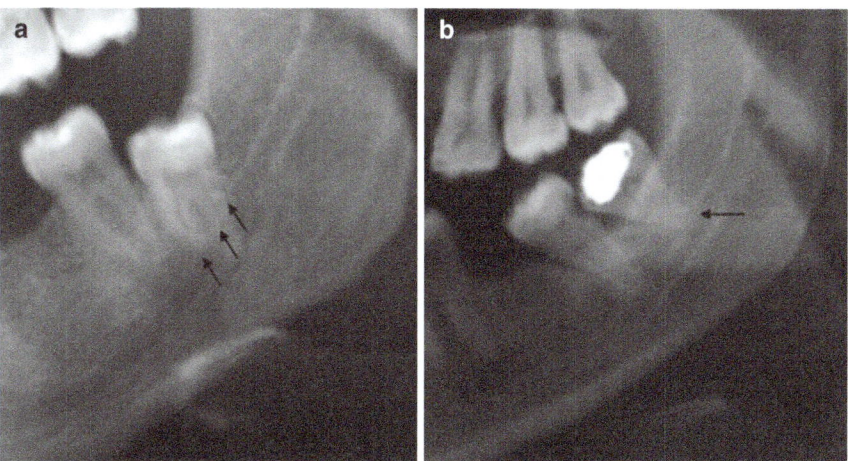

Fig. 2.23 In (**a**) the cortical of the mandibular canal (indicated by *arrows*) is detectable, even if projectively superimposed to the dental element. In (**b**) the cortical turns out to be focally deleted in correspondence to the radicular axis of 3.8 (indicated by *arrow*)

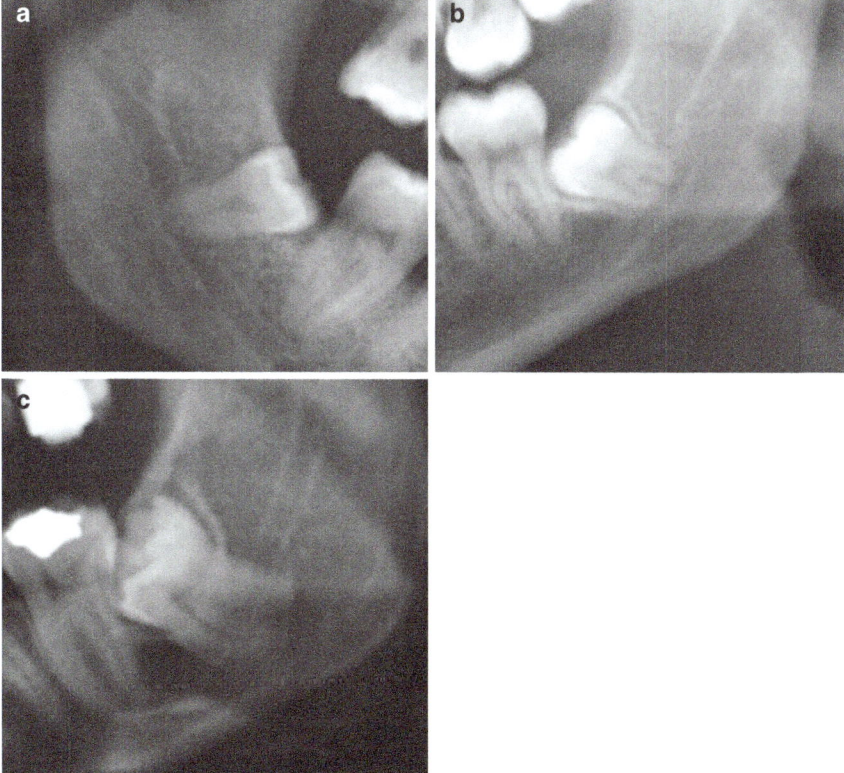

Fig. 2.24 (**a–c**) 'Critical' relations between the inclusive elements and the mandibular canal. In c 3.8 turns out to be a triradicular tooth. In all three cases disappearance of the mandibular canal's cortical occurs, which is indicative of the adjacency between the latter and the inclusive teeth

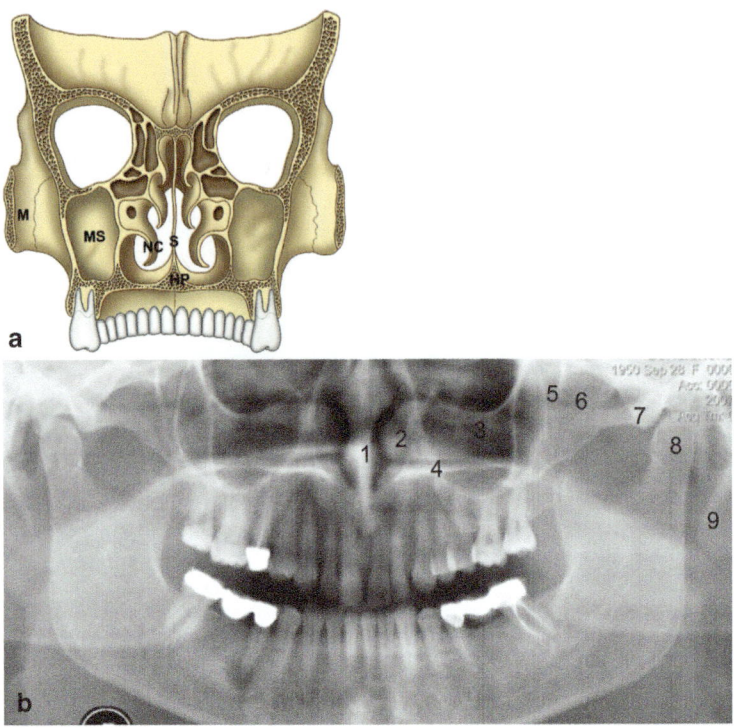

Fig. 2.25 (**a**) Schematic diagram which illustrates the main anatomical structures of the facial bones which are visible in OPT: *M* malar bone, *MS* maxillary sinus, *NC* nasal cavity, *S* nasal septum, *HP* hard palate. (**b**) Radiologic representation of the main anatomical structures visible in OPT: *1* nasal septum, *2* nasal cavity, *3* maxillary sinus, *4* hard palate, *5* pterygopalatine fossae, *6* pterygoid apophysis, *7* zygomatic arch, *8* mandibular condyle, *9* styloid apophysis

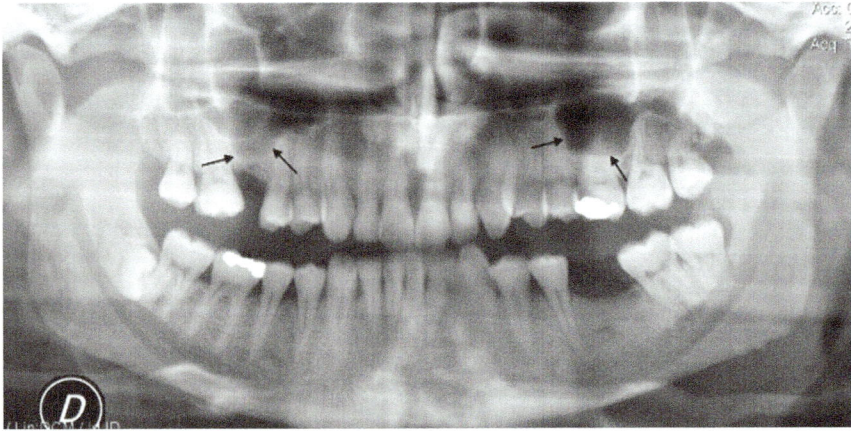

Fig. 2.26 Anatomical variation due to abnormal downward expansion of the maxillary sinuses (indicated by *arrows*). This situation can sometimes simulate the presence of radicular cysts

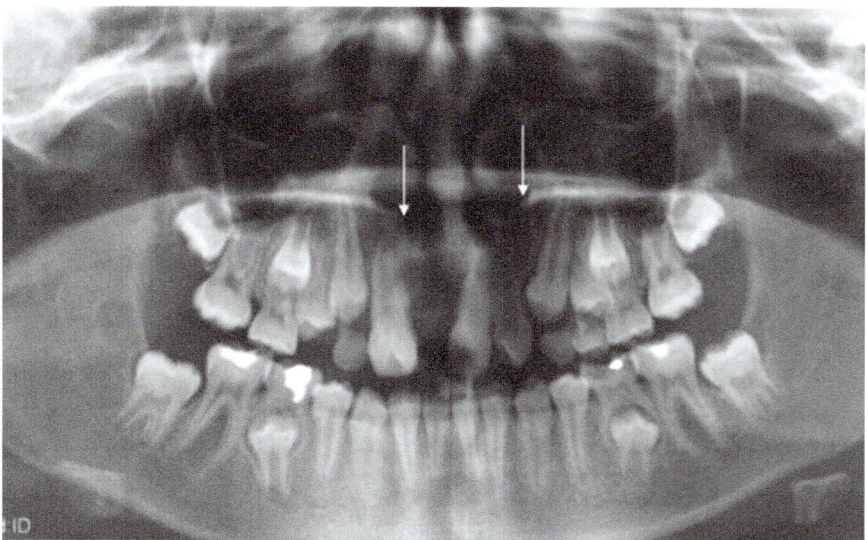

Fig. 2.27 The image shows palatoschisis. The *arrows* indicate the schisis margin affecting the hard palate

Fig. 2.28 Dysmorphic and rudimental dental element (indicated by *arrow*) which is inclusive in the left maxillary sinus

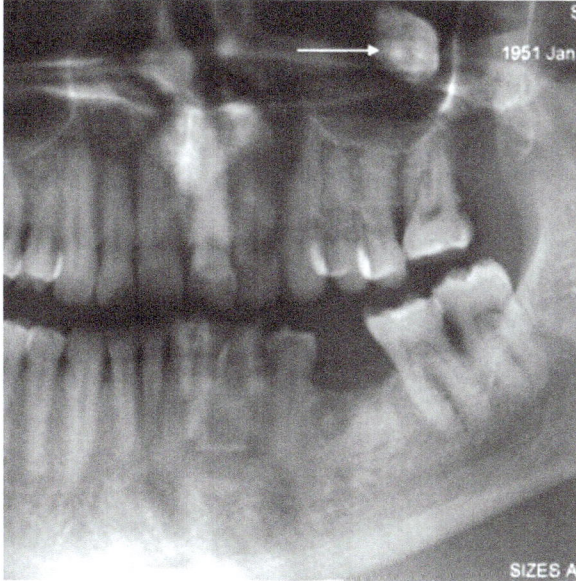

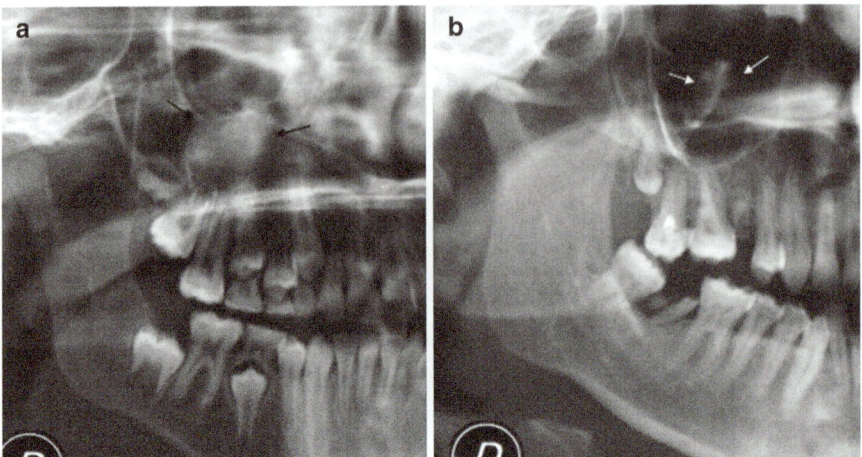

Fig. 2.29 (**a, b**) The image shows two cases of osteoma in the maxillary sinus (indicated by *arrows*)

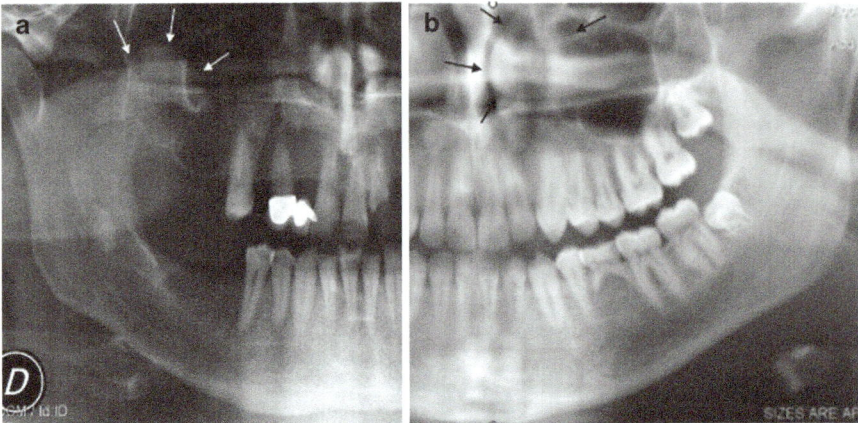

Fig. 2.30 (**a**) Mucous retentive cyst (indicated by *arrows*) of the right maxillary sinus. (**b**) Opacity, projecting itself into the maxillary sinus, due to the transport shadow of the inferior turbinate bone (indicated by *arrows*), which must not be confused with an endosinusal cystic lesion

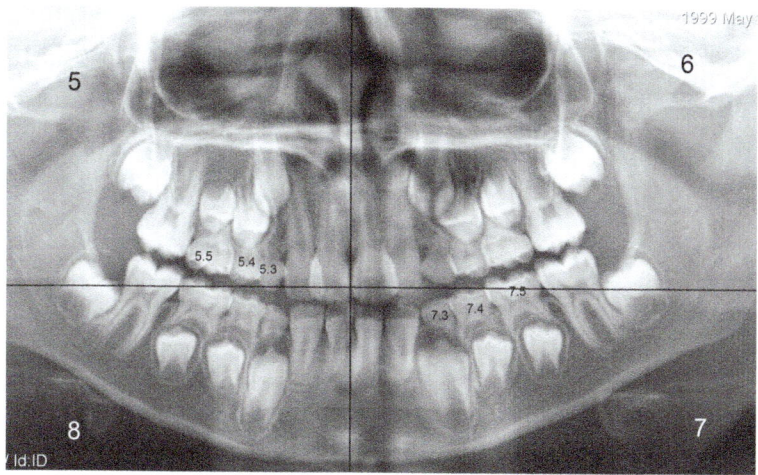

Fig. 2.31 Scheme showing the detection and the denomination of the deciduous elements

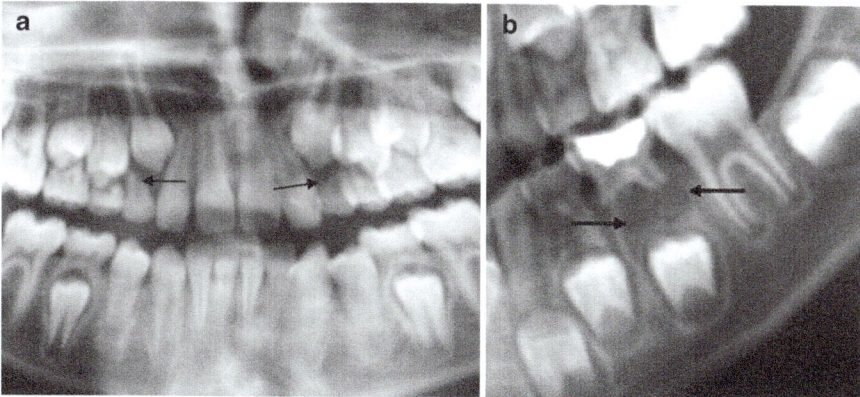

Fig. 2.32 (**a**) Physiological apicolysis (indicated by *arrows*) of the deciduous superior canines. (**b**) Pathological apicolysis in paediatric age due to flogistic periapical area of bone resorption (indicated by *arrows*) of a deciduous element

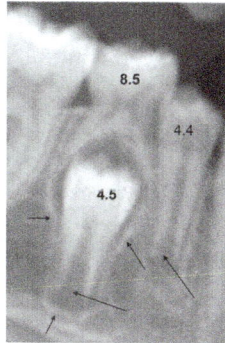

Fig. 2.33 Characteristic deciduous aspect of the inferior right deciduous second premolar (8.5). The correspondent permanent element (4.5) is in phase of dehiscence and it is possible to detect the alveolar or dental sac (indicated by *short arrows*). Both 4.4 and 4.5 typically present incomplete radicular axis with a wide apical foramen (indicated by *long arrow*)

Fig. 2.34 The image shows 4.3 and 4.4 in phase of dehiscence. The *long arrows* indicate the radiolucency which identifies the remains of the enamel organ

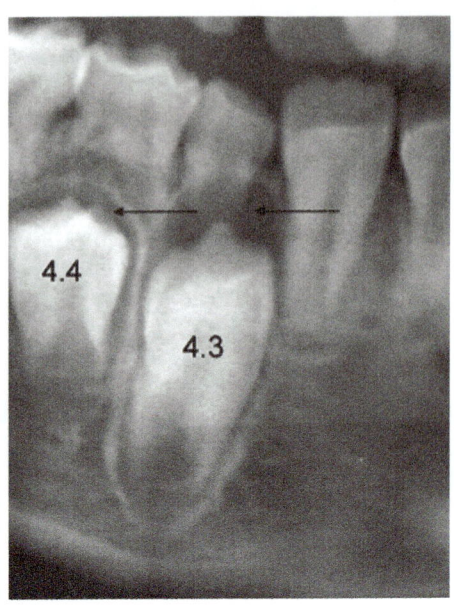

Suggested Reading

Barr JH, Stephen RG (1980) Dental radiology. Saunders, Philadelphia

Buchanan LS (2012) Everything's changed except the anatomy! Dent Today 31(9):100, 102, 104–105

Dharmar S (1997) Locating the mandibular canal in panoramic radiographs. Int J Oral Maxillofac Implants 12:113–117

Kim MS, Yoon SJ, Park HW, Kang JH, Yang SY, Moon YH, Jung NR, Yoo HI, Oh WM, Kim SH (2011) A false presence of bifid mandibular canals in panoramic radiographs. Dentomaxillofac Radiol 40(7):434–438

Langlais RP, Langland E, Nortje CJ (1995) Diagnostic imaging of the jaws. Williams & Wilkins, Baltimore/Philadelphia

Langland OE, Langlais R, Mc David W, Del Baso A (1989) Panoramic radiology, 2nd edn. Aufl, Lea & Febiger, Philadelphia

Maestre-Ferrín L, Carrillo-García C, Galán-Gil S, Peñarrocha-Diago M, Peñarrocha-Diago M (2011) Prevalence, location, and size of maxillary sinus septa: panoramic radiograph versus computed tomography scan. J Oral Maxillofac Surg 69(2):507–511

Park JH, Srisurapol T, Tai K (2012) Impacted maxillary canines: diagnosis and management. Dent Today 31:62, 64–66; quiz 68–69

Pria CM, Masood F, Beckerley JM, Carson RE (2011) Study of the inferior alveolar canal and mental foramen on digital panoramic images. J Contemp Dent Pract 12(4):265–271

von Arx T, Hänni A, Sendi P, Buser D, Bornstein MM (2011) Radiographic study of the mandibular retromolar canal: an anatomic structure with clinical importance. J Endod 37(12): 1630–1635. Epub 2011 Oct 26

White SC, Pharoah MJ (2000) Oral radiology: principles and interpretation. Mosby, St Louis

Part II

Elementary Radiographical Semeiotics and Pathological Terminology

The aim of the following section is to describe the main and more common detectable alterations in OPT, with particular regard to the elementary semeiotic elements and to the terminology used in medical reports.

It must be considered that, in the majority of cases, the diagnosis is basically dependent on clinical evaluation, as OPT is essentially an integrative and supporting technique to the odontostomatologue's actions.

It is also to say that the subdivision of the different pathological fields in separate chapters, even if useful from the didactic and expositive point of view, appears to be artificial. This is because in the majority of cases, the alterations tend to coexist together in a more or less significant way.

Pathological events which are detectable in OPT can be basically recognised as follows:

- Alterations of number, orientation, seat, morphology, width and structure of the dental element
- Caries
- Periapical alterations
- Alterations of the periodontal apparatus
- Focal lesions of maxillaries
- Alterations of the mandibular canal

Alterations of Number, Orientation, Seat, Morphology, Width and Structure of the Dental Element

3

This chapter includes numerous entities which can be characterised by a significant clinical impact or conversely are detectable in a functionally normal masticatory apparatus.

Of particular concern is the topic regarding the tooth anomalies which are correlated to errors of the development.

The field also comprises alterations of number, position, morphology, width and structure.

Number Anomalies

As previously explained, in the adult there are 32 permanent teeth. These are preceded by the 20 deciduous dental elements in evolutionary age subjects.

A number anomaly can occur in defect (**hypodontia**), in case of one or more teeth missing (**agenesis**) and in excess (**hyperdontia**), for the presence of one or more **supernumerary elements**.

Agenesis can be detected both in adult and paediatric age subjects.

However, in both cases, it is related to permanent dental elements.

Agenesis is a quite frequent event when limited to one or more dental elements; conversely, total agenesis or **anodontia** turns out to be extremely rare.

The dental elements affected by such anomaly are the second premolar teeth, the lateral incisors teeth and the third premolar teeth (Figs. 3.1, 3.2 and 3.3).

Dental agenesis, while more often detected in adults, is more important to be radiologically diagnosed in paediatric age subjects. In the latter, in fact, if a permanent dental element is clinically recognised as missing, the differential diagnosis includes both agenesis and a possible delay or **missed tooth eruption**. This may lead to the **inclusion** of the tooth (Figs. 3.4 and 3.5).

Another important point which can only be clarified radiologically is represented by the persistence of a deciduous element which is associated to the agenesis of the corresponding permanent dental element or to the presence of an inclusive permanent element (Figs. 3.6 and 3.7).

I. Pandolfo, S. Mazziotti, *Orthopantomography*,
DOI 10.1007/978-88-470-5289-5_3, © Springer-Verlag Italia 2013

However, particularly in the adult subject, the diagnostic finding regarding the lack of a dental element is fundamentally supported also by the anamnestic-clinical criterion. Sometimes, the radiographical characteristics of an **extraction site** can be useful to orientate the differential diagnosis between agenesis and the results of a previous dental avulsion (Fig. 3.8).

Structures of odontogenic origin must not be considered in the field of supernumerary teeth. These structures are often contained in maxillaries, which are in surplus when compared with the normal dental elements. However, due to their particular morphological characteristics, they are included in the topic of odontomas, which will be discussed in a later chapter.

The presence of supernumerary elements can pertain to the permanent dentition and, more rarely, to the deciduous one, with their prevalence in the superior arch (Fig. 3.9).

Although the phenomenon can occur in extremely variable and unpredictable ways, it must be noted that some of its manifestations turn out to be typical and well recorded clinically.

These manifestations include the so-called mesiodens. This is a small dental element, sometimes rudimental, typically situated between the central incisors in the median or paramedian region. It is characterised by a conoid or caniniform aspect (Figs. 3.10, 3.11 and 3.12).

On occasion, the caniniform aspect of the mesiodens is not present. In such circumstance, the element can appear variously dysmorphic (Fig. 3.13).

An error of interpretation can be committed when an inclusive canine tooth with a marked mesiodistal inclination (therefore close to the median line) is confused with a paramedian mesiodens.

In such a scenario, the detection of the correspondent deciduous element turns out to be decisive and clarifying (Fig. 3.14).

The so-called fourth molar is given rise to when supernumerary teeth occur. It is represented by an element with a very variable morphology (it can be a perfect developed tooth or a rudimental and/or hypoplastic tooth germ). It can be variably adjacent to the third molar, and it often has an altered orientation.

The phenomenon seems to be more frequent in the superior arch (Figs. 3.15, 3.16 and 3.17).

Even if it is characterised by a certain recurrence in its morphological aspects, its classification is always difficult. Indeed, it is not rare to observe unpredictable situations characterised by various complexity (Fig. 3.18).

The detection of possible supernumerary dental elements only assumes importance if they interfere with the planning of orthodontic and implantological treatments. Moreover, it can represent an obstacle to the correct eruption of the adjacent dental elements (Fig. 3.19).

To conclude, it must be underlined that even if OPT plays a key role in the detection of supernumerary teeth, it turns out to be inadequate for their correct localisation (vestibular vs. lingual). This is due to its bidimensional method.

With this perspective, it is obviously more efficient to use either endoral radiogram with occlusal technique or CT.

Anomalies of Position, Orientation and Seat

The present paragraph considers those dental elements, which, in the context of dental arches, present an anomaly in position, related to complete or incomplete **bone inclusion** phenomena.

It appears evident that the concept of inclusion must always be considered in relation to the patient's age, as the inclusion also represents a normal and transitional event in dental development.

Anomaly in position includes the orientation of the dental element, which may have altered.

Therefore, it is possible to distinguish between the normally oriented, inclusive elements and those with altered orientation (Figs. 3.20 and 3.21).

Anomalies of orientation that occur on the frontal plane can be well demonstrated using OPT. Indeed, it defines the **mesioangular angulation** (crown directed towards the medial line) or **distoangular angulation** (crown orientated to the opposite side).

Sometimes, this alteration can achieve extreme grades, till the dental element is completely inverted, with apex and crown facing the opposite side (Figs. 3.22 and 3.23a, b).

Conversely, anomalies of orientation in lingual or vestibular direction must be assessed by endoral study with occlusal projection or by CT. This is due to the impossibility of OPT to evaluate the dental anatomy in tridimensional way.

The clinical significance of the aforementioned alterations is extremely variable. Indeed, their presence is not always pathological. However, they often have troublesome implications for the planning of orthodontic and implantological treatments. Moreover, they can cause damage to the surrounding dental elements (Fig. 3.24) and give rise to complications such as **cystic degeneration of the enamel organ** (addressed later) (Fig. 3.25).

Clinical and legal-medical order issues can be behind the surgical treatment of the third inclusive and displaced molars. This could be due to their pathological relationship with the mandibular canal (Fig. 3.26).

The finding of dental elements beyond the dental arch is embryologically and clinically different (e.g., in the context of a maxillary sinus). In such situations **dental dystopia**, which is quite rare, occurs (Figs. 3.27 and 3.28).

Anomalies of Morphology and Dimensions

The alterations of the dental element's morphology and width are mainly caused by errors in development of the dental follicle.

Not all the following conditions have the same significance and equal clinical importance. Indeed, some conditions are merely curiosities with no practical relevance.

Others can both influence the clinical-functional point of view and represent a problem in case of avulsive or implantological therapeutic interventions.

Alterations of Morphology

This topic includes a series of malformative situations which are quite rare and heterogeneous. They are grouped for necessity of nosographic order rather than any analogy with etiopathogenesis.

Some entities, such as **concrescence**, **gemination** or **taurodontism**, turn out to be very rare.

Others, such as **dental scoliosis**, are more frequent; therefore, they are characterised by a major clinical impact.

Finally, it must be noted that a lot of dental malformations, often extremely odd, are of difficult placement. Due to their extreme polymorphism, they tend to deviate from the well-encoded morphological models. Indeed, they can only be grouped for the presence of some analogies.

Concrescence

It is a condition characterised by the radicular fusion (therefore at the level of the cement) of two elements. Such elements present crowns which are more or less dysmorphic, but with a covering of independent enamel (Figs. 3.29 and 3.30a, b).

Gemination

In this situation there is a unique root axis and an attempted separation of the crown. This crown splitting may appear prominent or be simply a hint (Fig. 3.31a, b).

Dens in Dente

It is the dysmorphism related to an abnormal invagination of the epithelial sheath in the context of dental matrix. As a consequence, an aberrant element forms inside the tooth (Fig. 3.32a, b).

Taurodontism

It is the alteration of the tooth development. It is constituted by a wide and squat crown and the absence of a developed root axis line.

Such malformation presents a wide range of variations. Some of them are categorised only as **taurodontia** only for the analogy to the main model and for convenience of exposition (Fig. 3.33a, b).

Curvature and Dental Scoliosis

This anomaly turns out to be more frequent than the previous ones, and it is characterised by major clinical relevance. This is due to the fact that the presence of curvature in the roots or in the whole dental element can cause troubles in extraction procedures and in endodontic treatments.

Curvature can concern both normal-placed (Fig. 3.34) and inclusive teeth. Moreover, it can be associated with anomalies of seat and orientation. This can give rise to complex situations which have to be recognised and considered (Fig. 3.35a–c).

Alterations of Dimensions

The following paragraph includes two entities: **macrodontia** and **microdontia**.

Macrodontia
It is a condition which stems from an error of embryonic development (fusion of two dental follicles). This leads to the consequent formation of elements with dimensions superior to the norm.

Real macrodontia (Fig. 3.36) must not be confused with the apparent dimensional increase of a tooth in relation to the secondary projective distortion, for example, the increase of distance between the tooth and the detection plane (Fig. 3.37a, b).

Microdontia
It is the opposite condition to the previous one.

It is represented by a deficit of growth in the dental follicle. As the follicle completes its development process, it gives birth to a tooth of significantly reduced dimensions in respect to the adjacent teeth (Fig. 3.38a–c).

Alterations of the Structure

The alterations of the dental structure 'in defect' do not have much practical importance; as in most cases, they are related either to rare systemic syndromes, such as **amelogenesis imperfecta**, **dentinogenesis imperfecta**, or to rare diseases such as **fluorosis**, **avitaminosis**, and **congenital syphilis**.

A situation of exiguous practical relevance, to be considered merely a curiosity and occasionally detected by OPT, is represented by the resorptive structure alteration which can sometimes be detectable in the crown of inclusive elements.

This process, which affects both the enamel and the dentine component, is most likely to be associated to trophic tissue alterations, probably related to the inclusion state (Fig. 3.39a, b).

Instead, structural alterations 'in excess' convey another significance both for frequency and practical implications. Such alterations include **idiopathic hypercementosis**, which represents the entity of major relevance.

It is an abnormal accumulation of cement in the root axis line whose nature and origin are not totally comprehended.

Idiopathic hypercementosis must be distinguished from the secondary or **reactive hypercementosis**, which has been evaluated as an epiphenomenon of periodontal and alveolar flogistic processes (Fig. 3.40).

Idiopathic hypercementosis, in addition to entailing an increase of the root density, is also the cause of its variable and sometimes significant volumetric growth (Fig. 3.41a–d).

Therefore, such an event can determine relevant problems in the case of an extraction procedure and during the endodontic treatment, as it can be associated to the obliteration of the radicular canal.

To conclude this chapter, the existence of some other conditions must be remembered.

They are generically considered as 'malformative', but of scant practical interest.

They include **enamel pearls** (micronodular aggregates of enamel exterior to the tooth and adjacent to the root or the crown) and what is known as **denticles or pulp stone**. This is the presence of a granular deposit of calcareous material in the canal or in the pulp chamber (Fig. 3.42).

This last entity must obviously not be confused with dens in dente.

Image Gallery

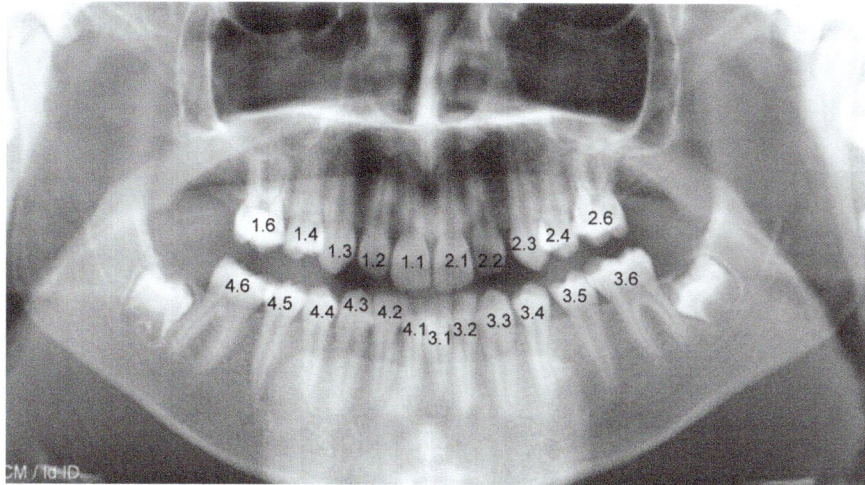

Fig. 3.1 Agenesis of 1.5 and 2.5. The permanent dental elements of the inferior arcade show normal anatomy

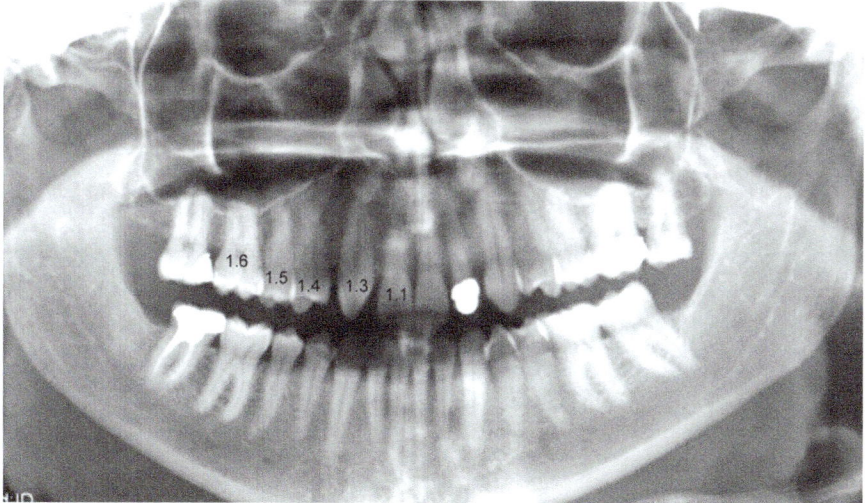

Fig. 3.2 Agenesis of 1.2

Fig. 3.3 Agenesis of 2.2 with persistence of the corresponding deciduous element (6.2)

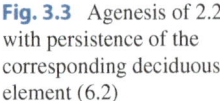

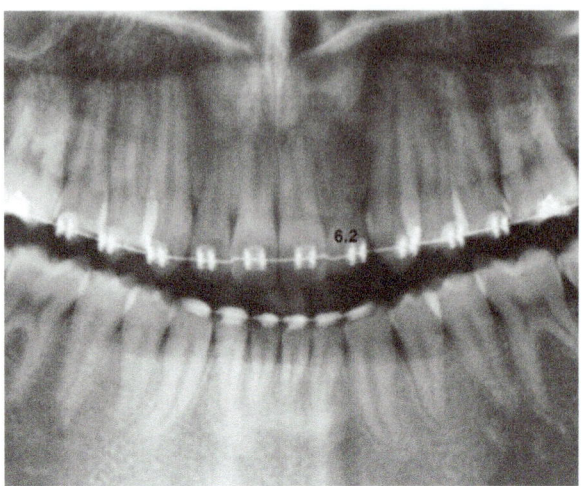

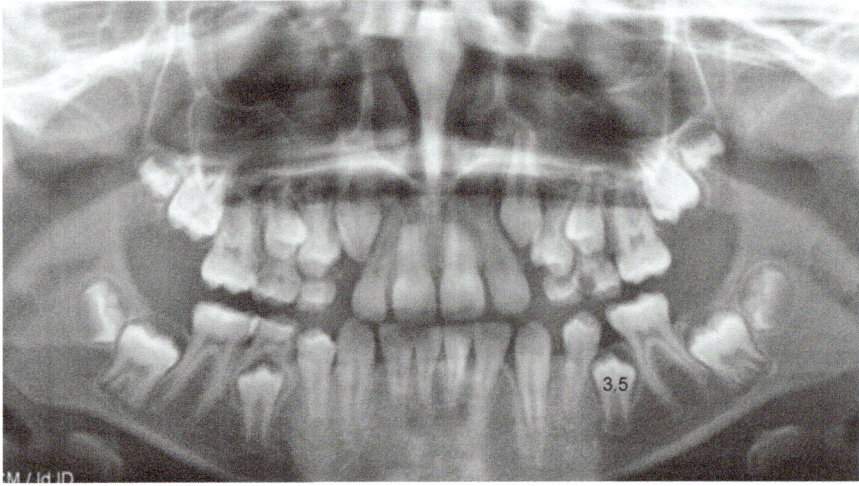

Fig. 3.4 The dental element which is not visible is not agenic but inclusive

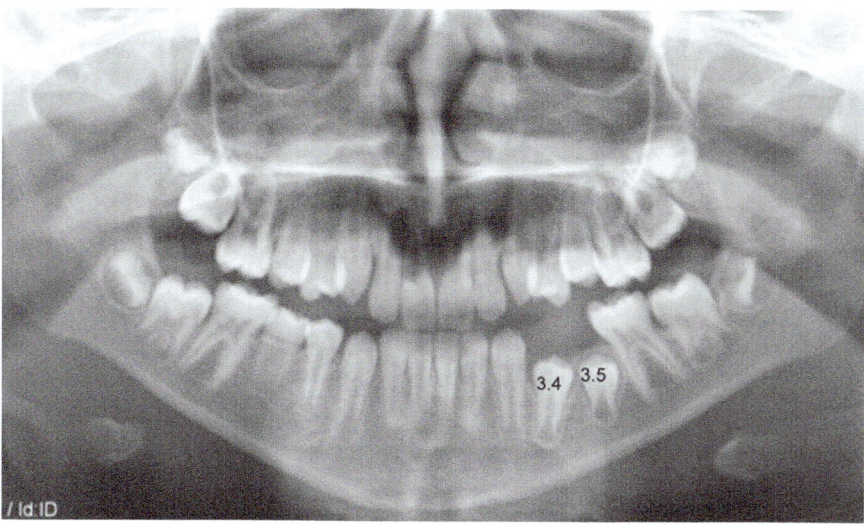

Fig. 3.5 3.4 and 3.5 are not visible under inspection as they are inclusive and not agenic

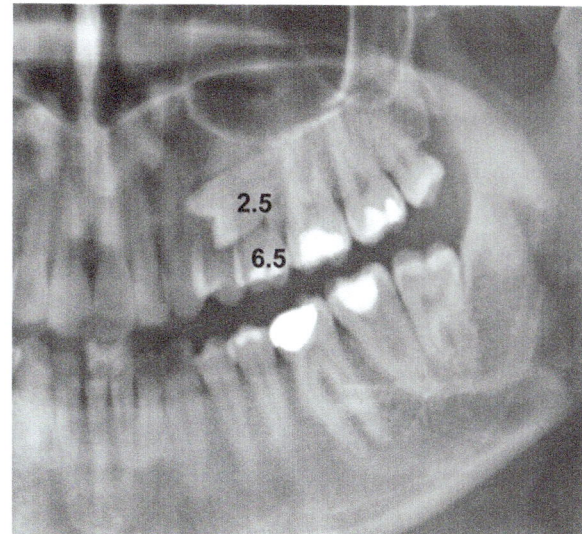

Fig. 3.6 Persistence of the deciduous element 6.5 with inclusion of the element 2.5 in mesiodistal angulation. The enlargement of 2.5 indicates that the latter is farther from the detection plane with respect to the adjacent elements (therefore it is located in palatal seat)

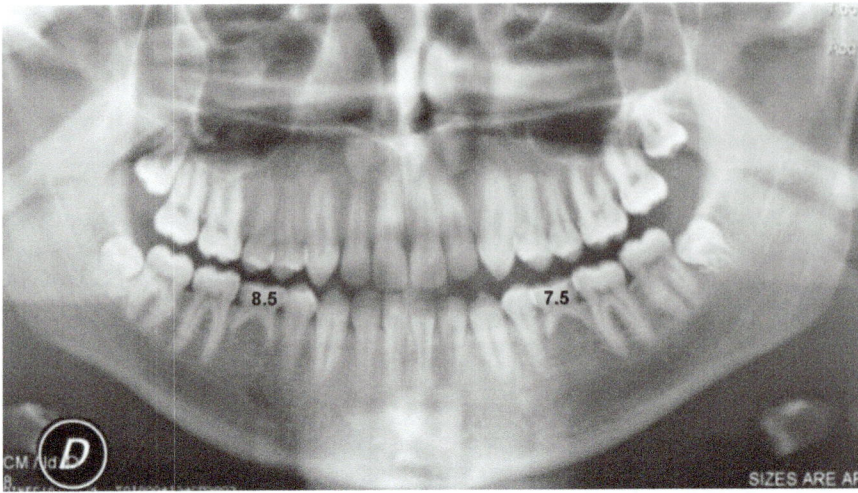

Fig. 3.7 Persistence of the deciduous elements 7.5 and 8.5 with agenesis of the corresponding permanent elements

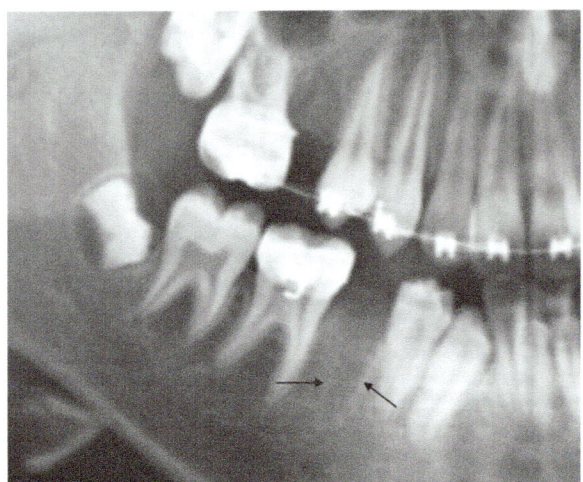

Fig. 3.8 The element 4.5 is not represented. The presence of the extraction site's vestigia (*arrows*) allows us to exclude agenesis

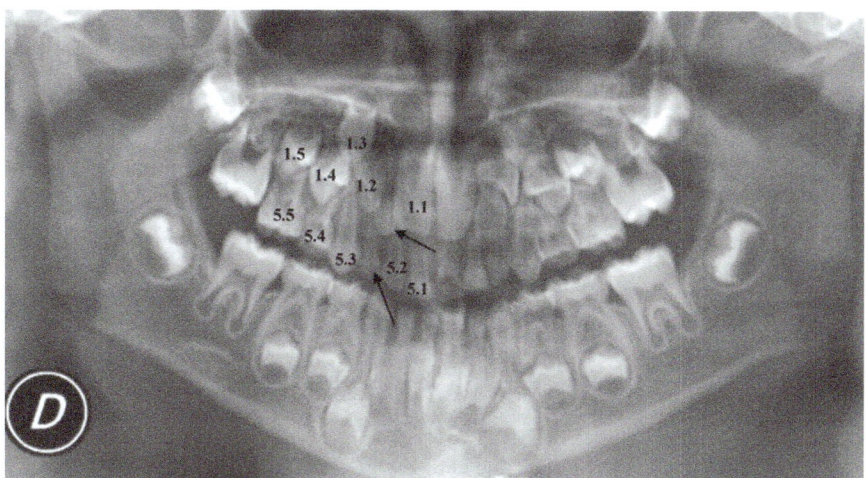

Fig. 3.9 Six deciduous and six permanent elements are detectable in the superior right hemiarch. The *arrows* indicate the surplus elements. A similar situation occurs in the superior left hemiarch

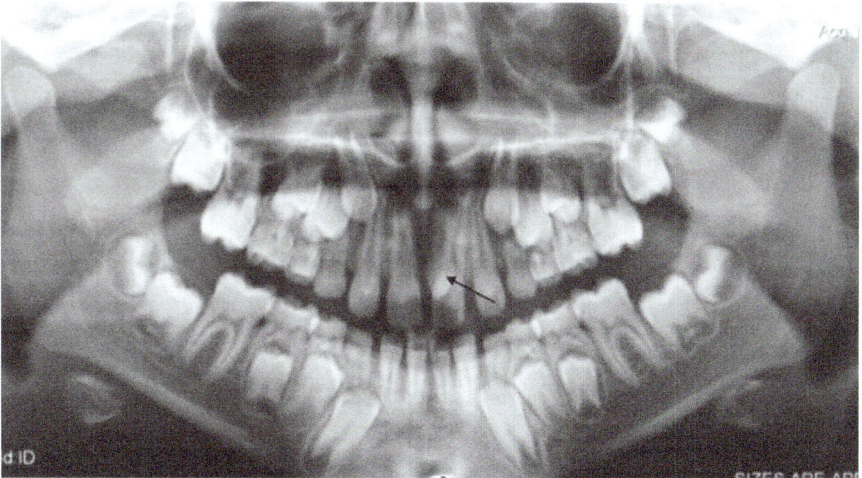

Fig. 3.10 Supernumerary caniniform element (indicated by *arrow*) between the superior median incisors (mesiodens)

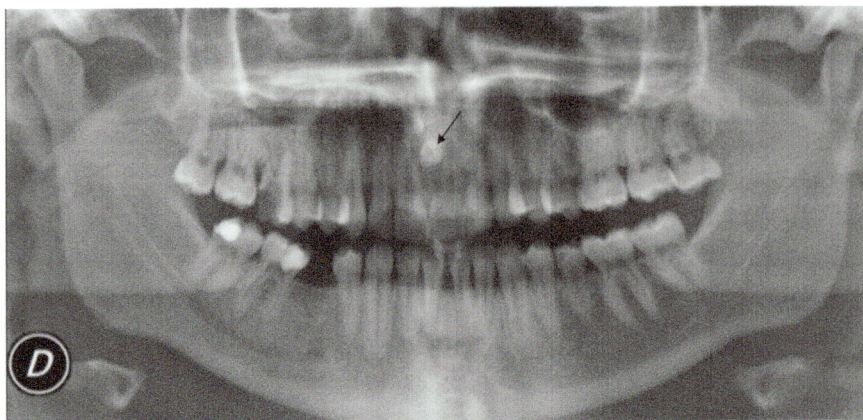

Fig. 3.11 Another type of mesiodens with rudimental aspect (indicated by *arrow*)

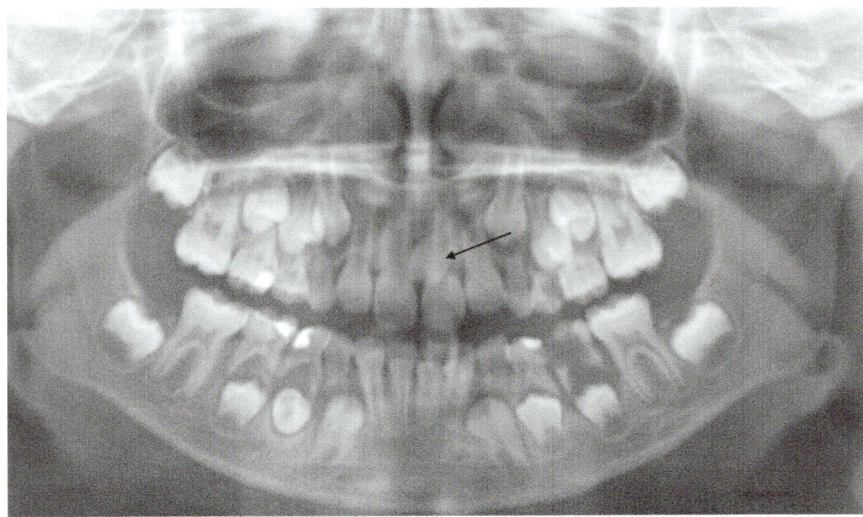

Fig. 3.12 Another mesiodens variation (indicated by *arrow*)

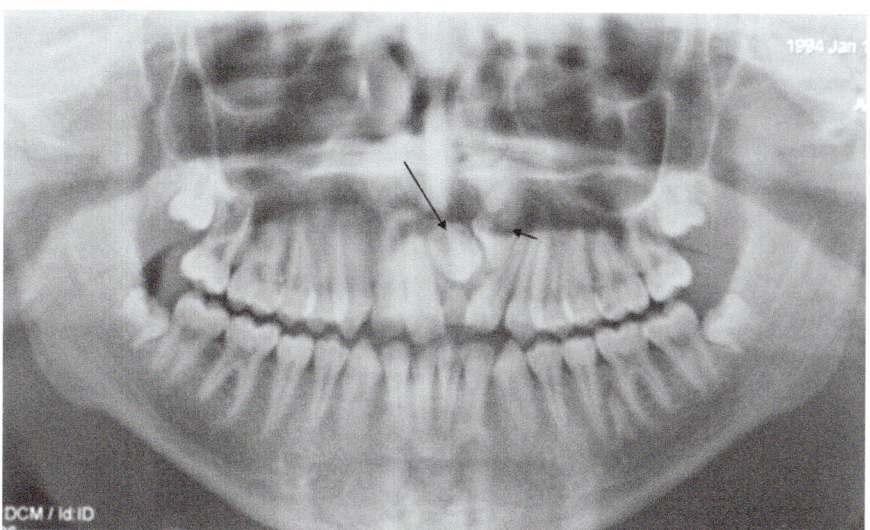

Fig. 3.13 Marked dysmorphic mesiodens (indicated by *long arrow*) which has impeded the eruption of the median superior left incisor (*short arrow*)

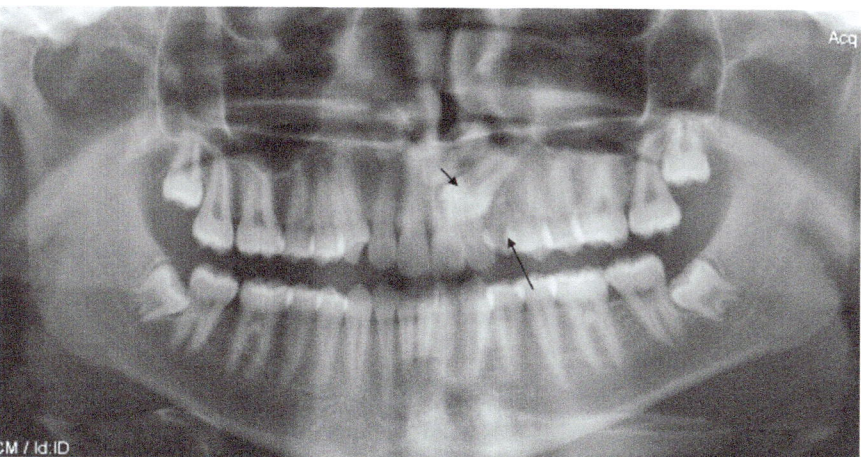

Fig. 3.14 The element 2.3 is inclusive and has a mesiodistal inclination (it is indicated by *short arrow*). This situation must not erroneously be confused with the presence of a mesiodens in paramedian seat. It is known to be an inclusive canine as persistence of the corresponding deciduous element (indicated by *long arrow*) occurs

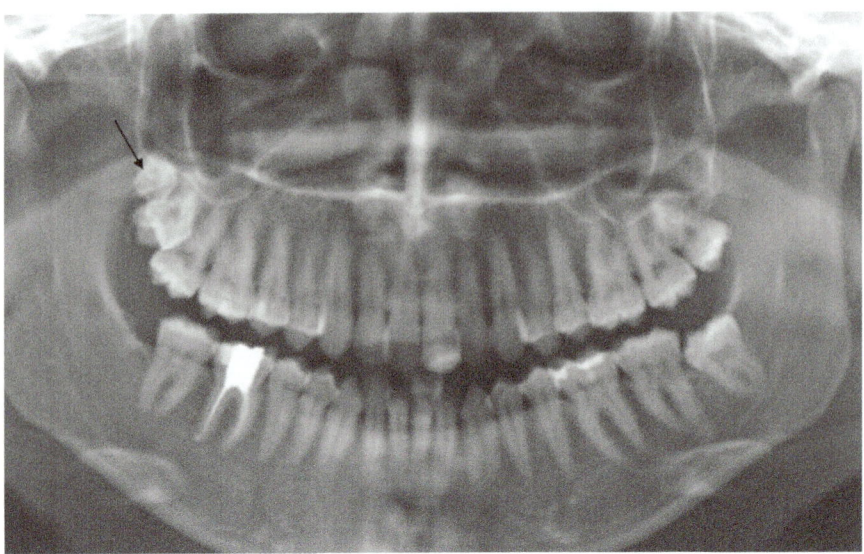

Fig. 3.15 Fourth inclusive and rudimental molar (indicated by *arrow*)

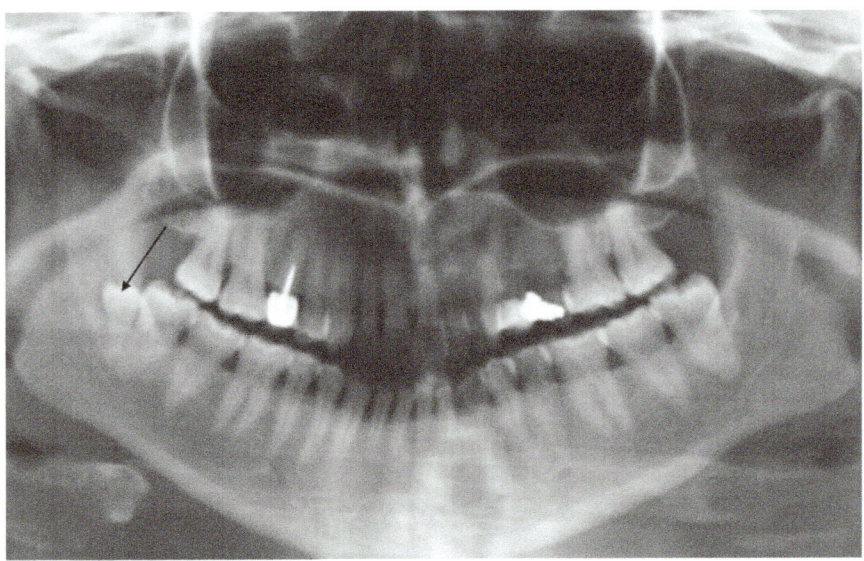

Fig. 3.16 Inclusive and normally formed fourth molar (indicated by *arrow*)

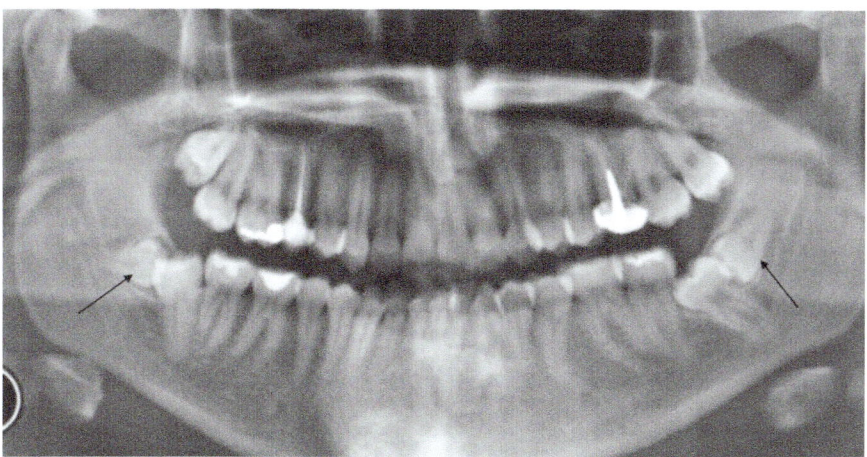

Fig. 3.17 Fourth molars which are inclusive, normally formed but with mesiodistal orientation (they are indicated by *arrows*)

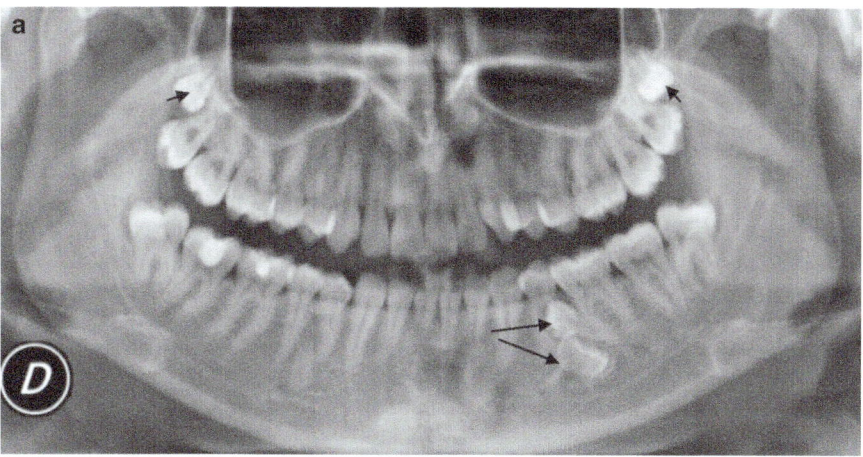

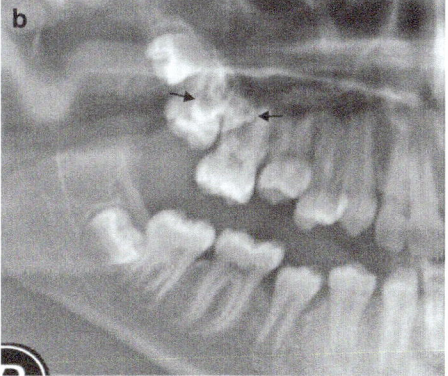

Fig. 3.18 (**a**) Complex case of supernumerary teeth showing fourth molars in the superior arcade (indicated by *short arrows*) and two inclusive elements (indicated by *long arrows*) in the inferior left maxillary, one of which is clearly a supernumerary tooth. (**b**) Supernumerary rudimental and dysmorphic element (indicated by *arrows*) which is inclusive between 1.6 and 1.7

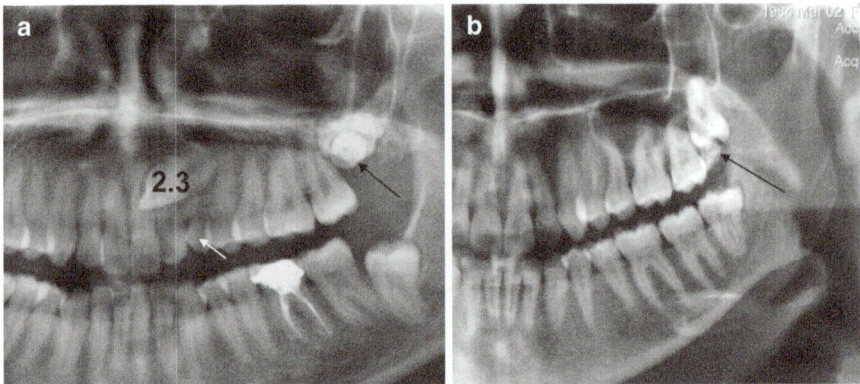

Fig. 3.19 (**a**) Rudimental supernumerary element (indicated by *long arrow*) which is opposed to the occlusal surface of 2.8. As a consequence, the element, which is inclusive in medio-distal inclination, has its eruption blocked. Persistence of the corresponding deciduous element (indicated by *short arrow*) also occurs. (**b**) Another rudimental supernumerary denticle (indicated by *arrow*) which impedes the eruption of 2.3

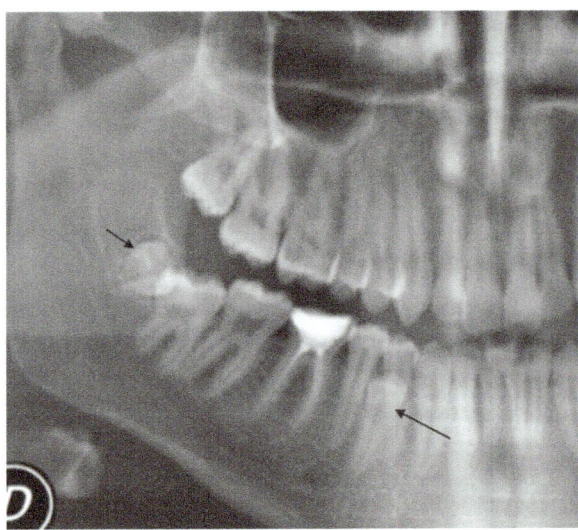

Fig. 3.20 4.4 is inclusive (indicated by *long arrow*) with persistence of the permanent element. A fourth molar is also present (it is indicated by *short arrow*)

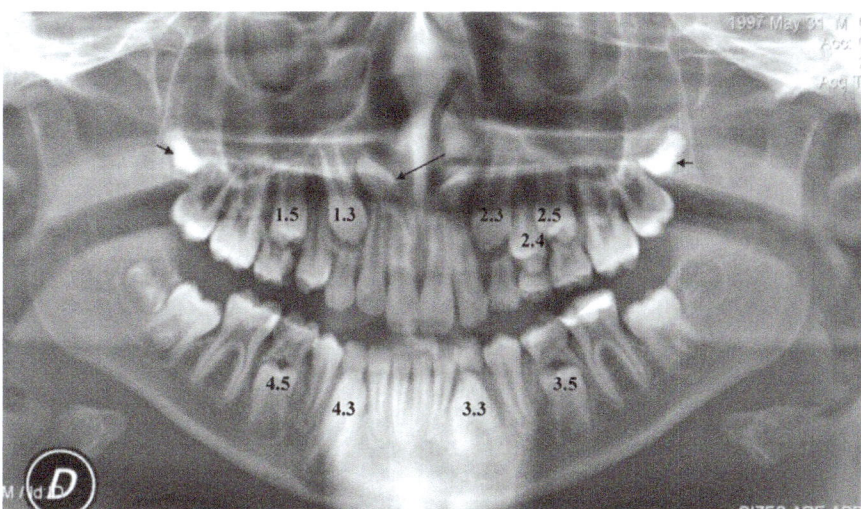

Fig. 3.21 Multiple permanent inclusive elements with normal orientation and deciduous elements regularly represented in a 13-year-old patient. In view of the age, the situation cannot be considered normal. Conversely, the inclusion of the eighth teeth (indicated by *short arrows*) is congruent with the age. Presence of the mesiodens (indicated by *long arrow*) is detectable, too

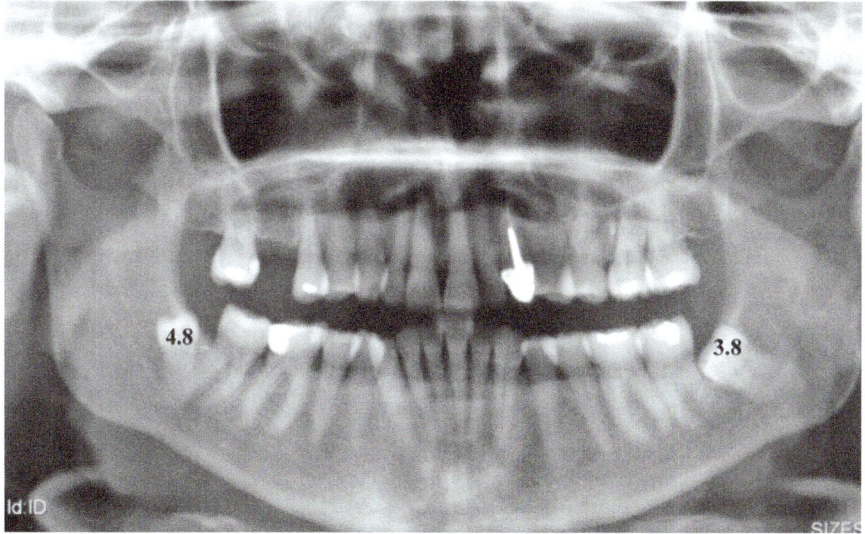

Fig. 3.22 3.8 is inclusive and in a slight mesiodistal angulation. 4.8 is inclusive and in a gentle distomesial angulation

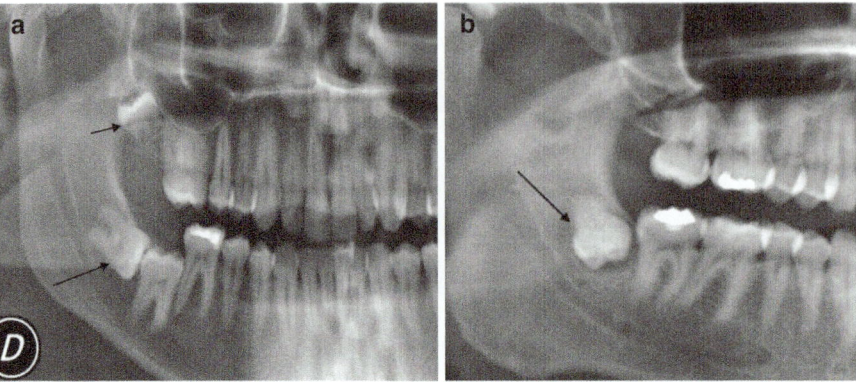

Fig. 3.23 Different and altered orientation in inclusive elements. (**a**) 4.8 in mesiodistal angulation (indicated by *long arrow*). 1.8 with inverted orientation (indicated by *short arrow*). (**b**) 4.8 inclusive and with inverted orientation (it is indicated by *arrow*)

Fig. 3.24 4.8 is normally erupted and in mesiodistal angulation. It is characterised by erosion due to the impact of the adjacent element in the cementoenamel junction (indicated by *arrow*)

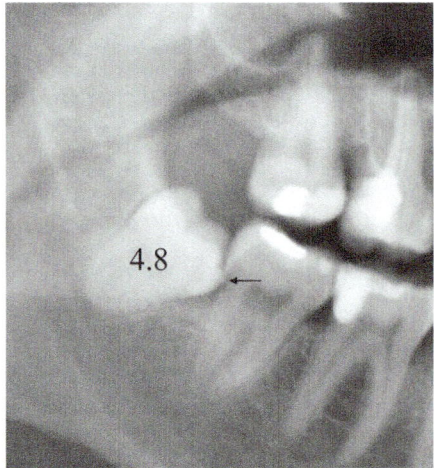

Fig. 3.25 4.3 is inclusive and shows an initial cystic evolution of the enamel organ's remains (it is indicated by *arrows*)

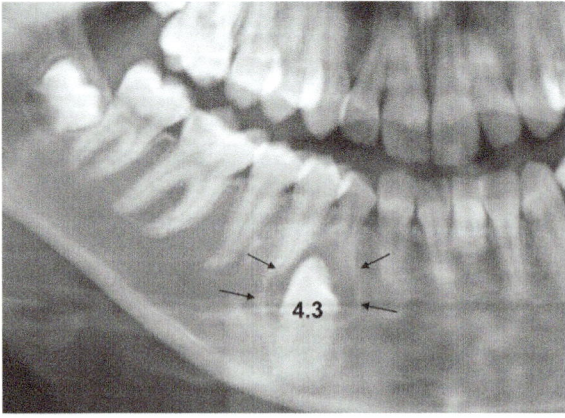

Fig. 3.26 3.8 is inclusive. Contiguity rapports with the mandibular canal (indicated by *arrows*) expose the latter to the risk of iatrogenic damage

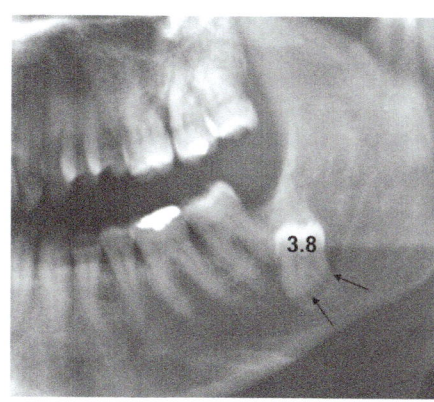

Fig. 3.27 Two supernumerary elements (indicated by *arrows*) in maxillary dystopia

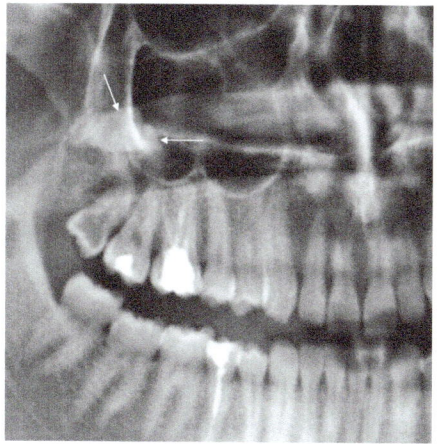

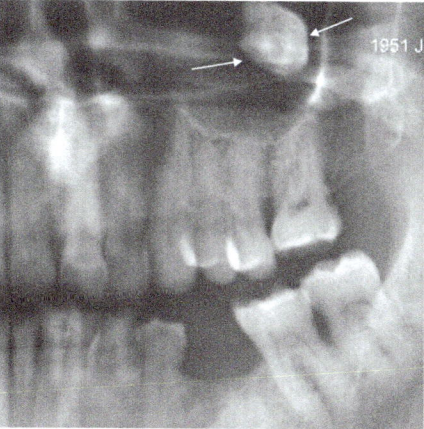

Fig. 3.28 Rudimental and dysmorphic element in maxillary dystopia (it is indicated by *arrows*)

Fig. 3.29 Scheme illustrating the phenomenon of concrescence. Each crown germ presents its enamel covering. Radicular fusion occurs

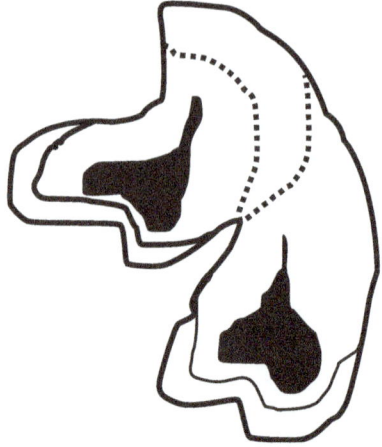

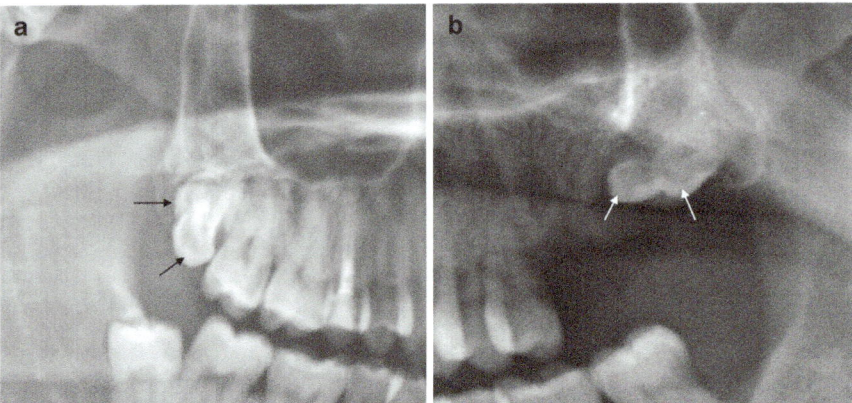

Fig. 3.30 (**a, b**) Two cases of concrescence. Each crown germ presents its enamel covering (indicated by *arrows*)

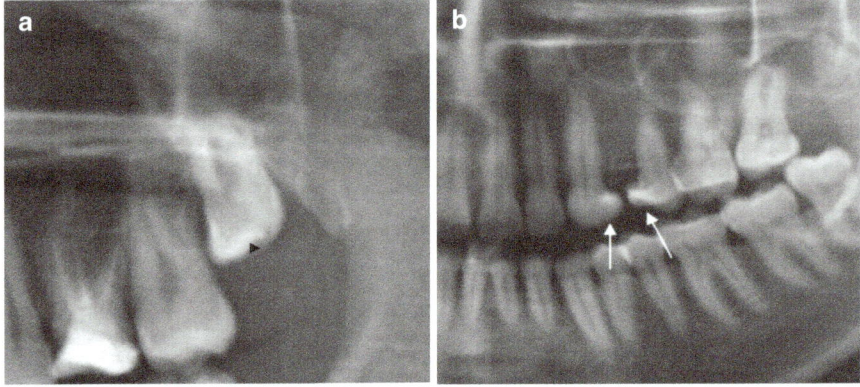

Fig. 3.31 (**a**) Malformed element with crown tending to gemination (*arrow head*). (**b**) Clear gemination of the crown of 2.3 and 2.5 (indicated by *arrow*). The element 2.4 is not represented as it is agenic

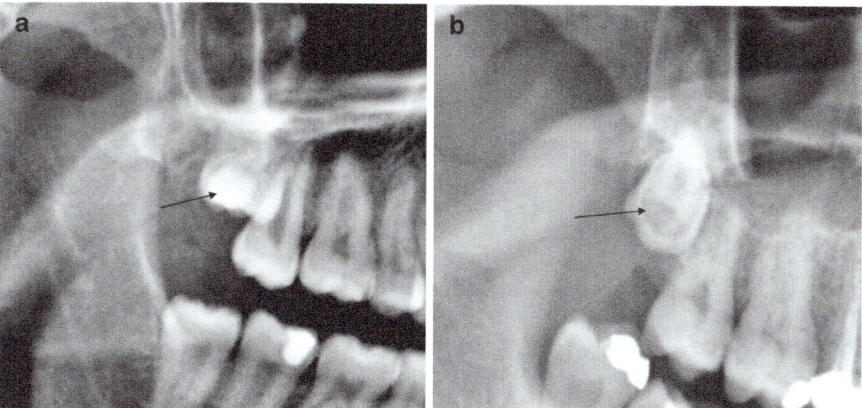

Fig. 3.32 (**a, b**) Two cases of dens in dente (indicated by *arrows*)

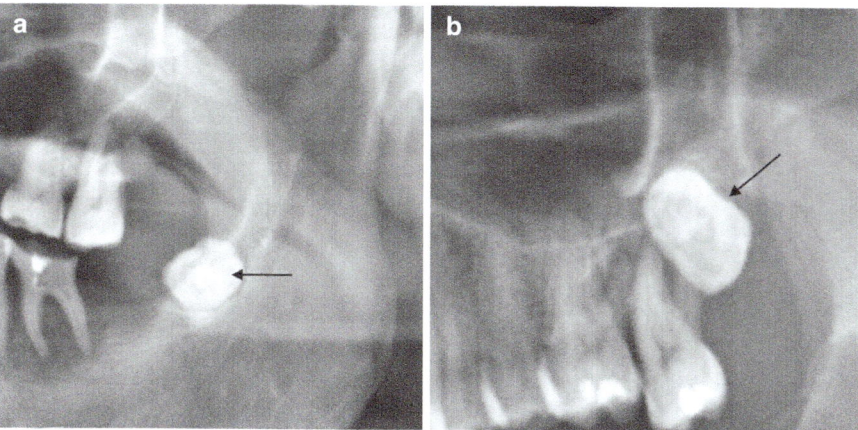

Fig. 3.33 (**a**) Typical element with taurodontic morphology characterised by wide and squat crown and absence of a developed root axis line (it is indicated by *arrow*). (**b**) Dysmorphic, squat element with scarce radicular representation (it is indicated by *arrow*) which, even if it is not typical, could be generally categorised as taurodontic

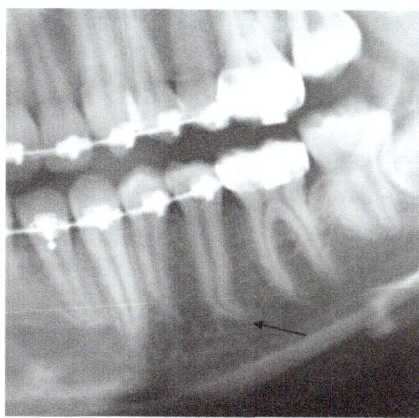

Fig. 3.34 Radicular curvature of the element 3.5 (it is indicated by *arrow*)

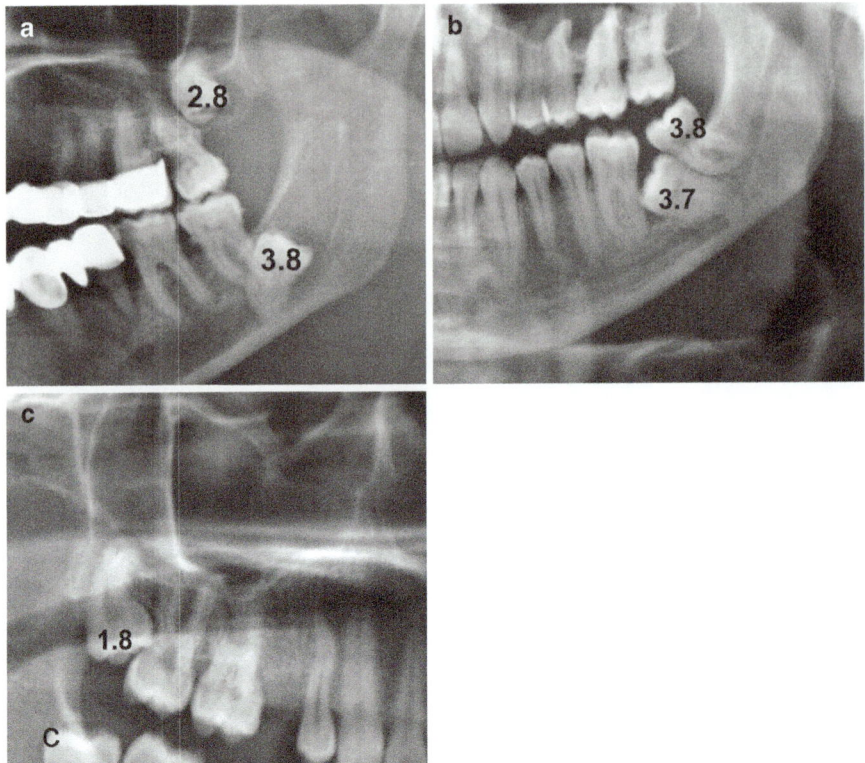

Fig. 3.35 (**a–c**) Various examples of curvature and dental scoliosis

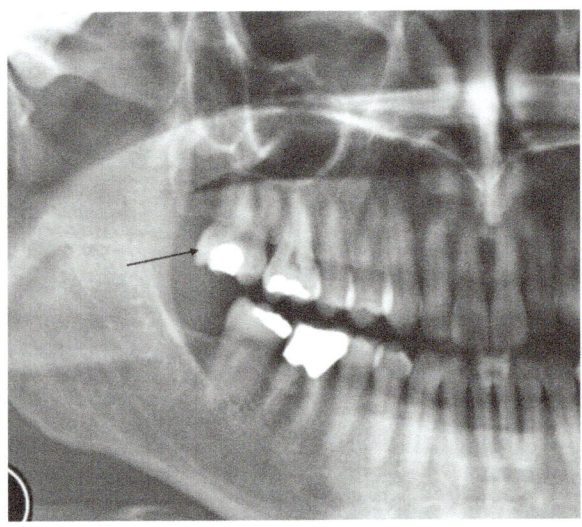

Fig. 3.36 Real macrodontia of the second molar (it is indicated by *arrow*)

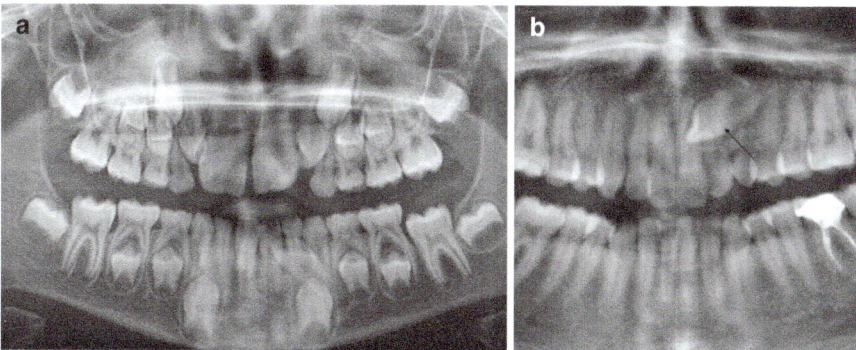

Fig. 3.37 (**a**) Real macrodontia of the central superior incisors. Only clinical observation is able to exclude a possible enlargement due to geometrical distortion (false macrodontia). (**b**) False macrodontia of an inclusive element (indicated by *arrow*). The tooth enlargement can be caused by its abnormal seat (palatal) which is farther from the detection plane

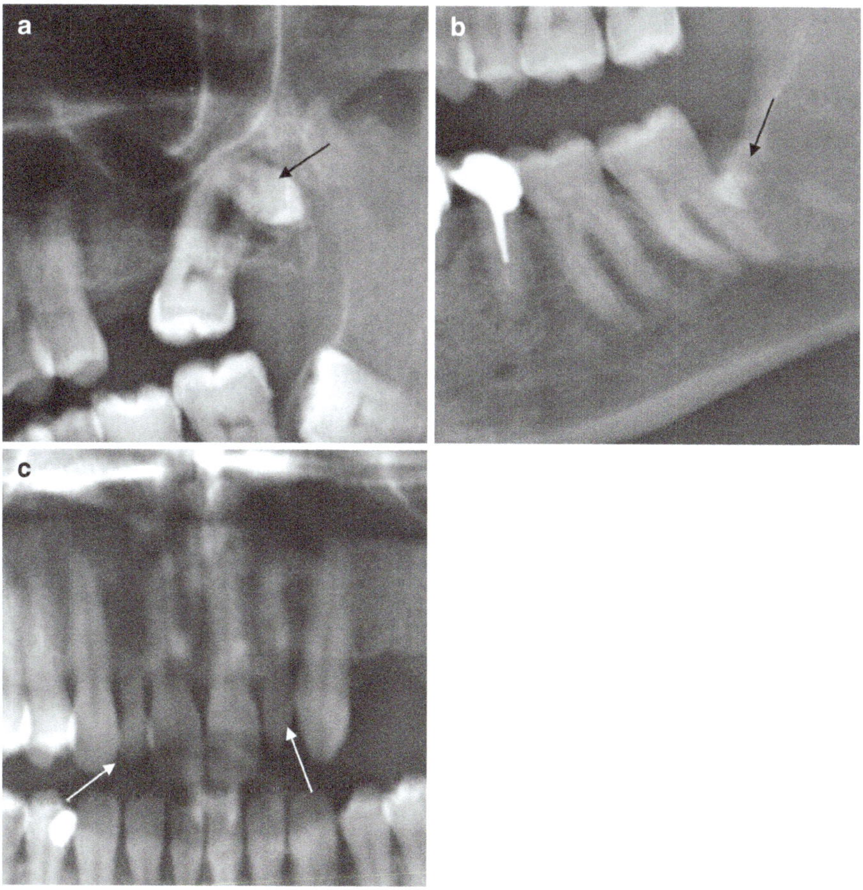

Fig. 3.38 (**a–c**) Three cases of microdontia (*arrows*)

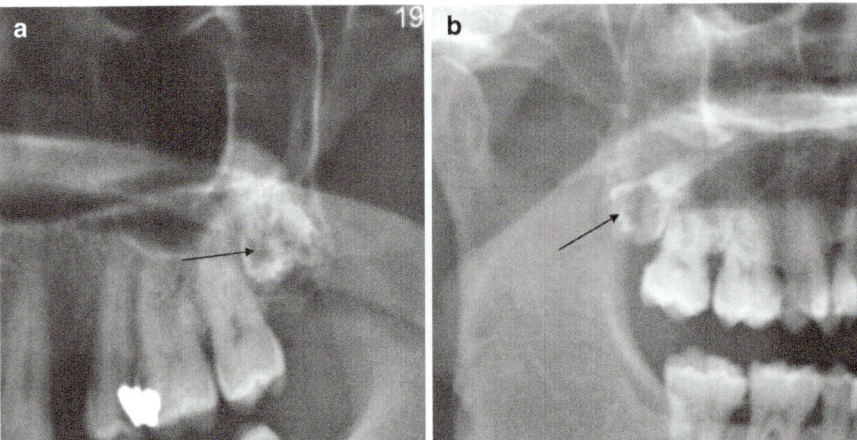

Fig. 3.39 (**a, b**) Structural alterations of inclusive elements' crown (they are indicated by *arrows*)

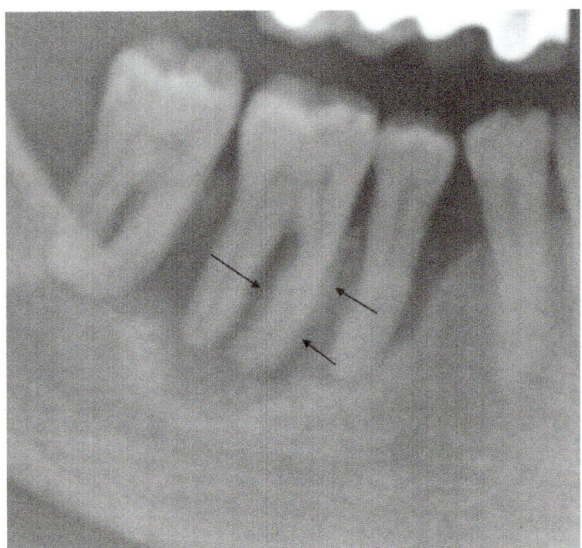

Fig. 3.40 Hypercementosis and enlargement of the mesial root of 2.6 (it is indicated by *arrows*) following alveolar flogosis phenomena

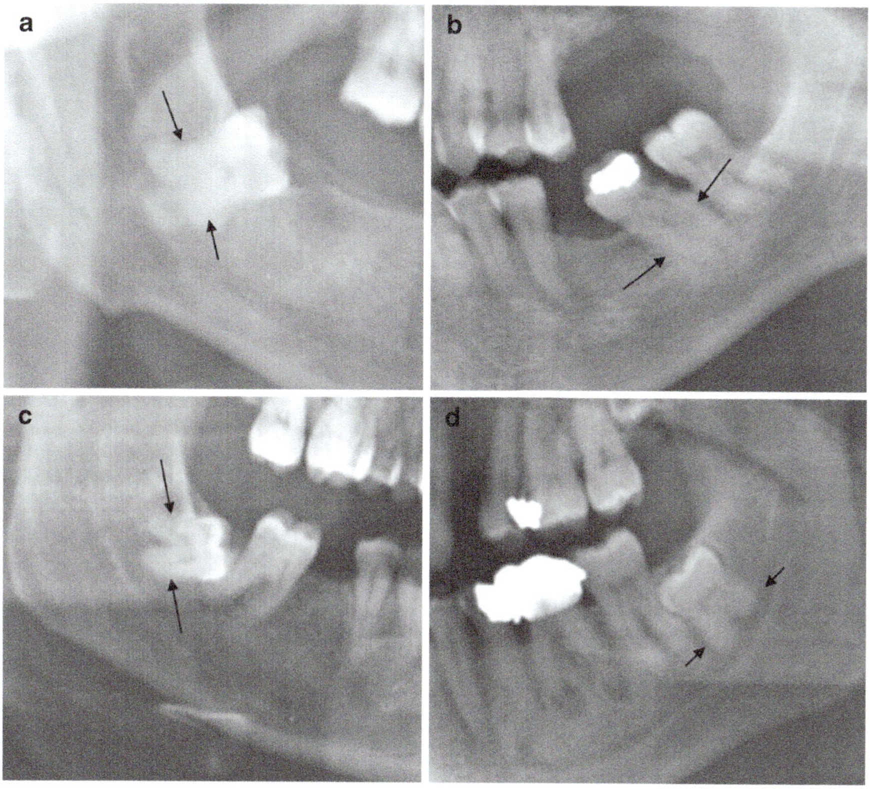

Fig. 3.41 (**a–d**) Different cases of idiopathic radicular hypercementosis (indicated by *arrows*)

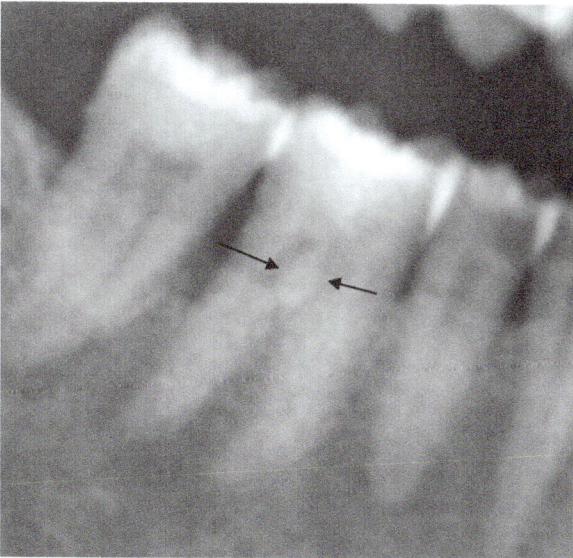

Fig. 3.42 Pulp stone (indicated by *arrows*) in the context of the pulp chamber

Suggested Reading

Benediktsdottir IS, Hintze H, Petersen JK, Wenzel A (2003) Accuracy of digital and film panoramic radiographs for assessment of position and morphology of mandibular third molars and prevalence of dental anomalies and pathologies. Dentomaxillofac Radiol 32(2):109–115

Celikoglu M, Bayram M, Nur M (2011) Patterns of third-molar agenesis and associated dental anomalies in an orthodontic population. Am J Orthod Dentofacial Orthop 140(6):856–860

Celikoglu M, Miloglu O, Kazanci F (2010) Frequency of agenesis, impaction, angulation, and related pathologic changes of third molar teeth in orthodontic patients. J Oral Maxillofac Surg 68(5):990–995

Dula K, Mini R, Van der Stelt PF, Buser D (2001) The radiographic assessment of implant patients: decision making criteria. Int J Oral Maxillofac Implants 16(1):80–88

Frederiksen NL (1995) Diagnostic imaging in dental implantology. Oral Surg Oral Med Oral Pathol Oral Radiol Endod 80(5):540–554

Langland OE, Langlais R, Mc David W, Del Baso A (1989) Panoramic radiology, 2nd edn. Aufl, Lea & Febiger, Philadelphia

Le T, Nassery K, Kahlert B, Heithersay G (2011) A comparative diagnostic assessment of anterior tooth and bone status using panoramic and periapical radiography. Aust Orthod J 27(2):162–168

Montasser MA, Taha M (2012) Prevalence and distribution of dental anomalies in orthodontic patients. Orthodontics (Chic) 13(1):52–59

Poyton HG (1980) Oral radiology. Williams & Wilkins, Baltimore

Sajnani AK, King NM (2012) The sequential hypothesis of impaction of maxillary canine – a hypothesis based on clinical and radiographic findings. J Dent Child (Chic) 79(1):34–39

Şekerci AE, Şişman Y, Ertaş ET, Gümüş H, Ertaş H (2012) Clinical and radiographic evaluation and comparison of six cases of fusion involving the primary dentition. J Dent Child (Chic) 79(1):34–39

Updegrave WJ (1963) Panoramic dental radiography. Dent Radiogr Photogr 36:75

Van Parys K, Aartman IH, Kuitert R, Zentner A (2012) Relationship between dental anomalies and orthodontic root resorption of upper incisors. Eur J Orthod 34(5):571–574. Epub 2011 Jul 10

Van Parys K, Aartman IH, Kuitert R, Zentner A (2011) Assessment of dental anomalies on panoramic radiographs: inter- and intraexaminer agreement. Eur J Orthod 33(3):250–255. Epub 2010 Aug 26

White SC, Pharoah MJ (2000) Oral radiology: principles and interpretation. Mosby, St Louis

Caries

4

Caries, or dental decay is a pathological destructive process which can affect all the components of the dental elements (enamel, dentine, cement), always in an irreversible way.

It is caused by a disturbance in the homeostasis existing between the floral bacteria (streptococcus, lactobacillus, etc.) and the local and systemic immune defences.

An increase in bacterial load or a reduction of the immune defences breaks this balance and determines the onset of caries. Caries is also furthered by the sugar fermentation activity performed by bacteria, with a consequent production of local hyperacidity. The latter has the effect of destroying the **hydroxyapatite** crystals and therefore the enamel integrity.

In the relevant literature, numerous studies show that radiological evaluation significantly (about 30–50 %) increases detection of caries lesions, with respect to the clinical examination.

While clinical evaluation plays a fundamental role in the diagnosis and in the evaluation of the extension of the caries lesion, it is clear that radiological examination, in a considerable percentage of cases, mainly plays a complementary role.

All of the literature concerning this topic shows different classification systems of caries, both on clinical and radiological basis.

Radiological categorisation of caries evaluates the effects on the enamel (whether in partial or full thickness), the dentine and eventually the pulp chamber.

With regard to this, it must be noted that such classifications derive from the evaluations of the endoral radiological examination which, as is known, is characterised by a resolution power which is superior to the OPT one.

As a consequence, the evaluation of caries through OPT suffers from some limitations, especially related to the quantification of damage.

From a practical point of view however, in orthopantomographic examination it is sufficient to distinguish between the damage of the enamel and the dentine's one and between the latter and a possible involvement of the pulp chamber.

This last eventuality gives rise to '**penetrating caries**' which, because of this contamination of the chamber, along with the pulp canal and its content, will result in a series of complications.

I. Pandolfo, S. Mazziotti, *Orthopantomography*,
DOI 10.1007/978-88-470-5289-5_4, © Springer-Verlag Italia 2013

A further progression of the damage, followed by a much wider affection of the crown, will give rise to so-called destructive caries, obviously easily detectable on the clinical point of view.

From the radiological point of view, caries, regardless of its evolutionary stage, presents itself as a radiolucent lesion which affects both the crown and the cementoenamel junction. Its morphology varies in relation to the projective conditions with which it is represented.

Indeed, it seems evident that carious lesions captured in profile will be characterised by sharply defined outlines and by a semilunar morphology. Conversely, frontally hit lesions, though maintaining the sharpness of their outlines, present a roundish morphology.

Finally, caries which, due to their position, are captured in three-quarter view present irregular morphology and blurred, badly definable outlines (Fig. 4.1a–c).

Depending on its localisation, caries must be distinguished into **occlusal, interproximal (or interstitial caries), palatal and vestibular caries**.

Occlusal caries originate at the level of the tooth's masticatory surface.

The caries are easily detectable with inspection, and radiological evaluation is useful to estimate the extent of their depth (Figs. 4.2a–c and 4.3a–c).

Occlusal caries develops in an area where the enamel presents maximum thickness. Consequently it is characterised by a later involvement of the pulp chamber when compared with other localisations.

Indeed, slow evolution allows the formation of the so-called reactive dentine which in turn contributes to further delay of this destructive process (Fig. 4.4).

Interproximal caries originate at the level of the contact surfaces between the elements. Therefore, they can appear both in the mesial side and in the distal side (Figs. 4.5a–c and 4.6a–d).

Interproximal caries are less detectable in radiographical examination as the interdental surfaces are less explorable than the other portions of the tooth.

The aforementioned carious localisations can simultaneously affect the interproximal surfaces of two adjacent elements, giving rise to opposed interproximal caries (**distal interproximal caries** and **mesial interproximal caries**). Such caries are often characterised by a different evolutionary stage (Fig. 4.7a–c).

In their pathogenesis, interproximal caries can show anatomical conditions favourable to development and progression of the pathological event.

In this scenario, caries which arise after the impact of an adjacent element with abnormal angulation appear to be paradigmatic (an event which occurs typically in situations of **disodontiasis of the third molars**).

Due to their pathological contact, also the presence of crown capsules and/or **excessive teeth fillings** can determine the appearance of carious lesions in the adjacent interproximal surface (Fig. 4.8a, b).

As the carious lesions affecting the tooth's vestibular and lingual surface are frontally hit by the incident beam, they are transferred onto the radiogram as radiolucent areas. Their morphology will be variously rounded, with neat or blurred outlines respective to the conditions of interface between lesion and healthy tissue, as well as the projective conditions. Lesions captured in three-quarter view, or otherwise not perfectly orthogonal to the incident beam, can present blurred outlines and irregular morphology.

It turns out to be evident that, due to the impossibility of representing the seat of the lesion in a tridimensional way, OPT is unable to distinguish between the vestibular and the lingual seat of the lesion (Fig. 4.9a–c).

For the same reasons, the involvement of the pulp chamber/canal is demonstrable, with major difficulties compared to interproximal and occlusal caries.

It is very clear that the distinction of the carious lesion based on its seat is quite artificial and is most often useful merely for descriptive and semantic aims.

Indeed, caries often affect more contiguous sub-seats, and in more advanced cases (destructive caries), they give rise to radiological representations in which the seat of origin is no longer traceable.

The most extreme case is represented by the complete destruction of the crown with the persistence of **radicular remains** only (Fig. 4.10a–c).

Some particular considerations are necessary with caries originating at the level of the cementoenamel junction.

This area represents a weak point due to its anatomical characteristics (junction line where the enamel and the cement are mutually located and where both sheaths present the minimum thickness). For this reason, it is one of the more frequent seats of caries onset.

The aforementioned anatomical feature explains why, at such level, caries of small dimensions can also lead to an early affection of the dentine (Fig. 4.11a, b).

Typically and for the same reason, the onset of caries at the level of the cementoenamel region can be characterised by a particular morphology indicative of so-called pit caries, characterised by a narrow orifice and by a wide expansion of the lesion deep into the dentine (Fig. 4.12).

Caries Complications

The carious lesion, if not treated, can cause damages both within the pulp and on the periodontal side.

In the first case, alterations will entail the flogistic and infective involvement of the dental pulp with ever more serious **pulpitis** phenomena ending with colliquative necrosis.

In such eventualities, the pathological process, through the apical foramen, can transfer itself to the surrounding area of the tooth, giving birth to a **periapical lesion** (topic treated in the following chapter).

From the radiological point of view, dental pulp alterations are not directly visible.

Conversely, it is possible to provide evidence of the so-called endodontic damage, expressed by the erosive phenomena within the internal pulp canal which itself appears irregularly widened (Fig. 4.13a–c).

Contrarily, in some cases, characterised by minor biological aggresiveness and chronic course, the pulp canal can be blocked by the production of reactive dentine, rendering it undetectable by radiological examination (Fig. 4.14).

However, we must note that such observation lacks specificity as the radiological non-detection of a pulp canal can also occur in a completely normal tooth or in the presence of primary or secondary hypercementosis.

The destruction of a periodontal ligament by a carious lesion (particularly if it originates in the neck region) causes the progression of the infection in the periodontal space, which, in some cases, creates a preformed course towards the apical region (Fig. 4.15a, b).

This last condition gives rise to **focal periodontitis** (topic that will be discussed also in Chap. 6).

Secondary or Recurrent Caries

Secondary caries or **recurrent caries** is a carious lesion which originates beneath a tooth filling or another possible covering device (a capsule, a bridge, etc.).

The role of radiology in the detection of such lesions typology, of difficult clinical identification, is evident.

Secondary caries appears as a radiolucent area interposed between the tooth and the radiopaque material of the filling and is characterised by an extremely variable morphology.

Indeed, it can assume the classic aspect of crateriform caries (Fig. 4.16a–d), or it can express itself only as a thin radiolucent line.

There is no doubt that in this last eventuality, the radiological diagnosis of secondary caries must be carefully made, as the aforementioned radiolucent line could simply be the expression of a weak adherence between the tooth and the reconstructive device, with or without the interposition of a restorative material, which is radiolucent, too (Fig. 4.17a–c).

Complications of untreated caries (both primary and secondary) include also pathological **dental fractures**. They are due to the loss of the normal biomechanical resistance of the tooth, and they can affect the crown, the roots or the whole dental element (Fig. 4.18a–d).

False Caries

To conclude this chapter, it must be emphasised that not all the radiolucent images involve the presence of caries. Indeed, they can be related to situations of other nature, which do not have pathological meaning and can be easily evaluated through direct observation.

In such a scenario, the image of false carious erosion is extremely characteristic. It is sometimes recognisable at the level of the cementoenamel junction and is caused by an optical effect generated by the extreme thinness which is characterised by the interface between the enamel and the cement in such seat (Fig. 4.19).

Another situation which can be misleading is represented by the presence of substance losses (both for treated caries and after traumatic lesions) repaired with radiolucent restorative material, which are not radiographically visible.

In such cases (which generally affect the front teeth), the radiological aspect of the lacunar images is quite characteristic for the sharpness of the outlines (Fig. 4.20).

However, the error can be easily avoided by visually checking the patient's denture.

Finally, **dental abrasions** and **dental fissures** must not be considered as caries.

Dental abrasions are caused by prolonged **occlusal trauma**, and for this reason they are always visible at level of the masticatory surface (Fig. 4.21a, b).

Dental fissures usually have iatrogenic origin. They can have a linear or triangular morphology, with sharp limits, representing the most significant differential semeiological element with respect to the real caries (Figs. 4.22a, b and 4.23).

Image Gallery

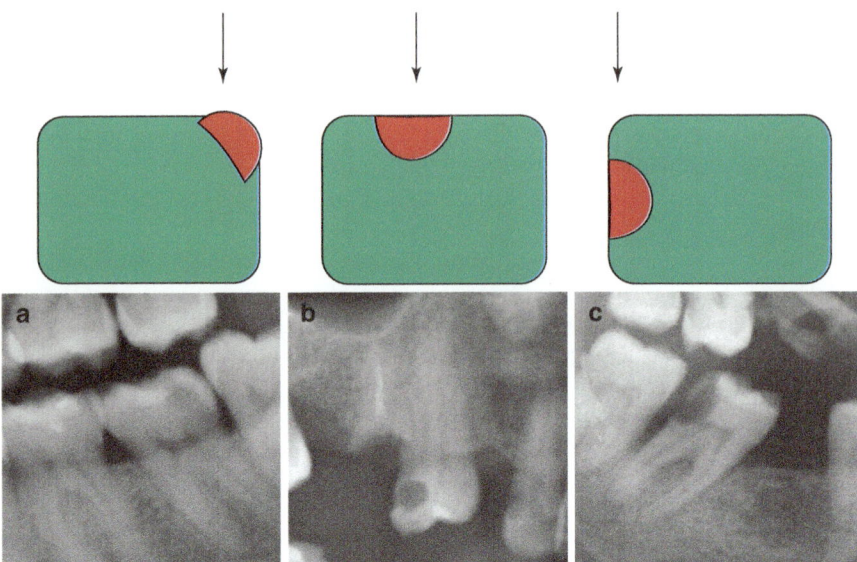

Fig. 4.1 Variations of the radiological morphology of the carious lesion in relation to the different projective conditions. (**a**) Caries captured in three-quarter view. (**b**) Caries captured frontally. (**c**) Caries captured in profile

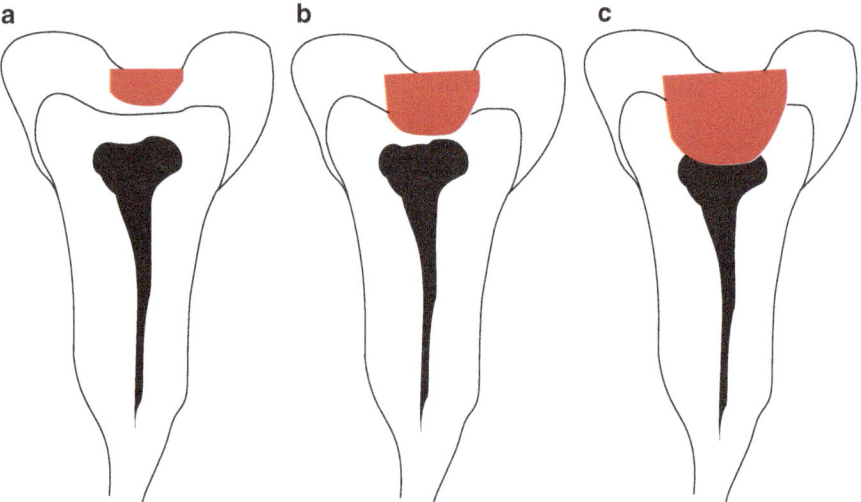

Fig. 4.2 Schematic diagram which illustrates the progression in depth of the occlusal caries. (**a**) Affection of the enamel. (**b**) Affection of the dentine. (**c**) Affection of the pulp chamber

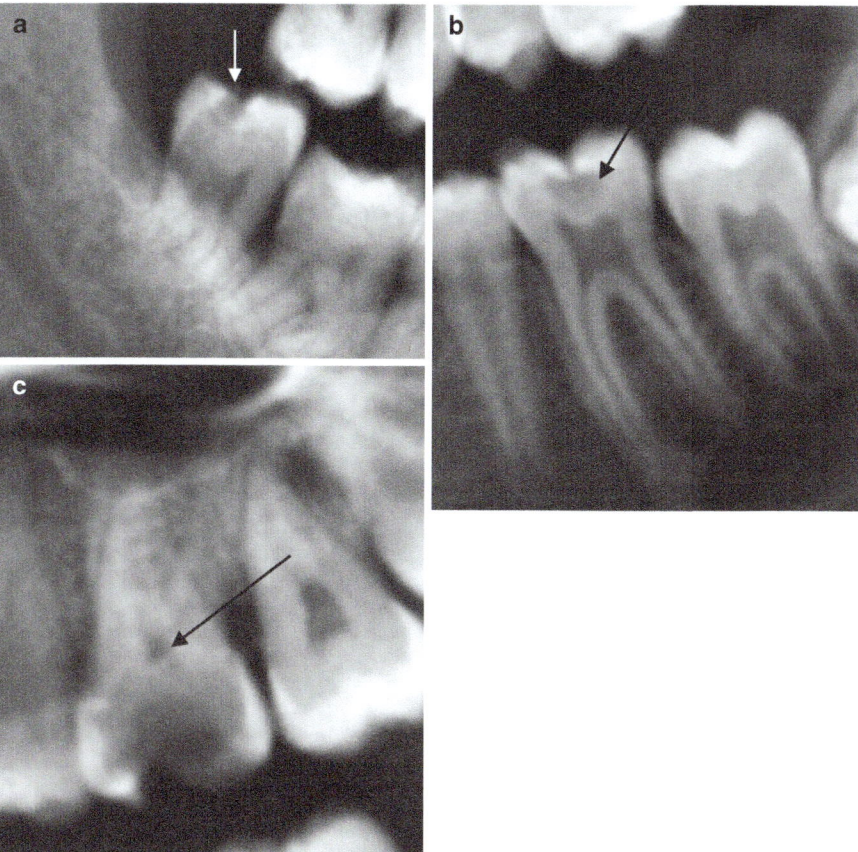

Fig. 4.3 Different evolutionary stages of the occlusal caries (indicated by *short arrows*). (**a**) The lesion is limited to the enamel. (**b**) The lesion extends itself towards the dentin. (**c**) The lesion affects the pulp chamber (directed by *long arrow*)

Fig. 4.4 Wide occlusal
caries (indicated by *arrow*)
separated from the pulp
chamber by a band of major
opacity (*arrowheads*),
expression of the presence of
reactive dentine

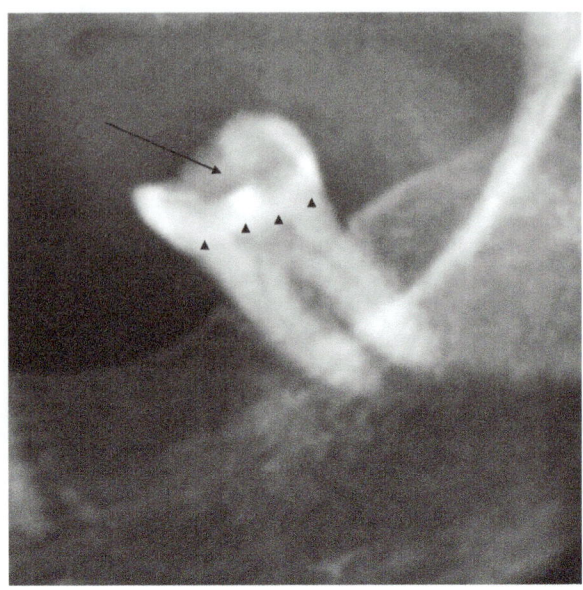

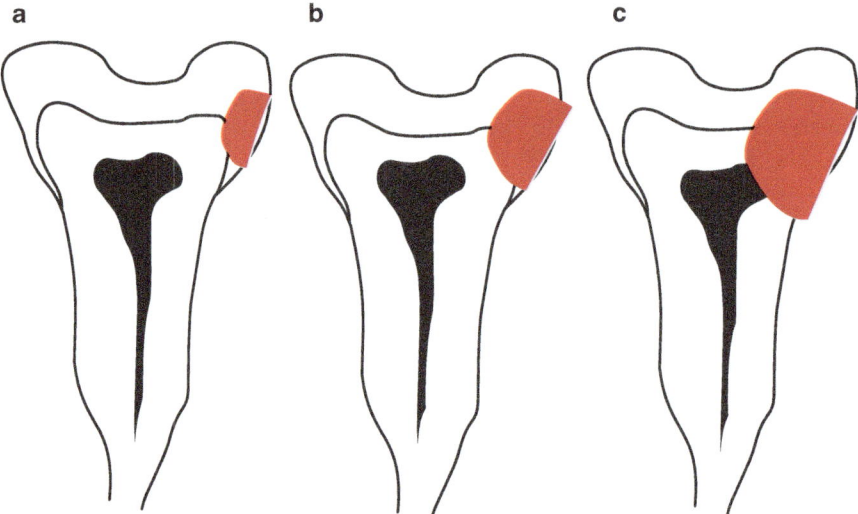

Fig. 4.5 Different evolutionary stages of the interproximal caries. (**a**) Affection only of the
enamel. (**b**) Affection of the dentine. (**c**) Affection of the pulp chamber

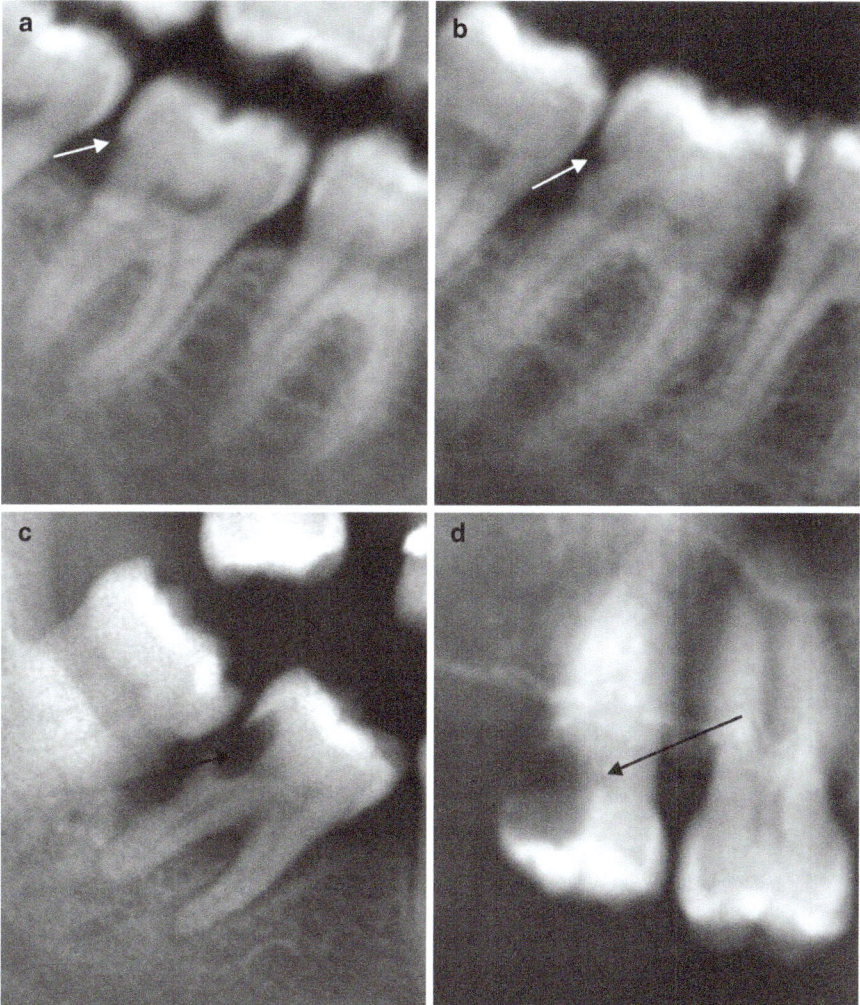

Fig. 4.6 Different evolutionary stages of the interproximal caries (indicated by *short arrows*). (**a**) Distal caries limited to the enamel. (**b**) Distal caries affecting only the dentine. (**c**) Affection in depth of the dentine. (**d**) Affection of the pulp chamber (indicated by *long arrow*)

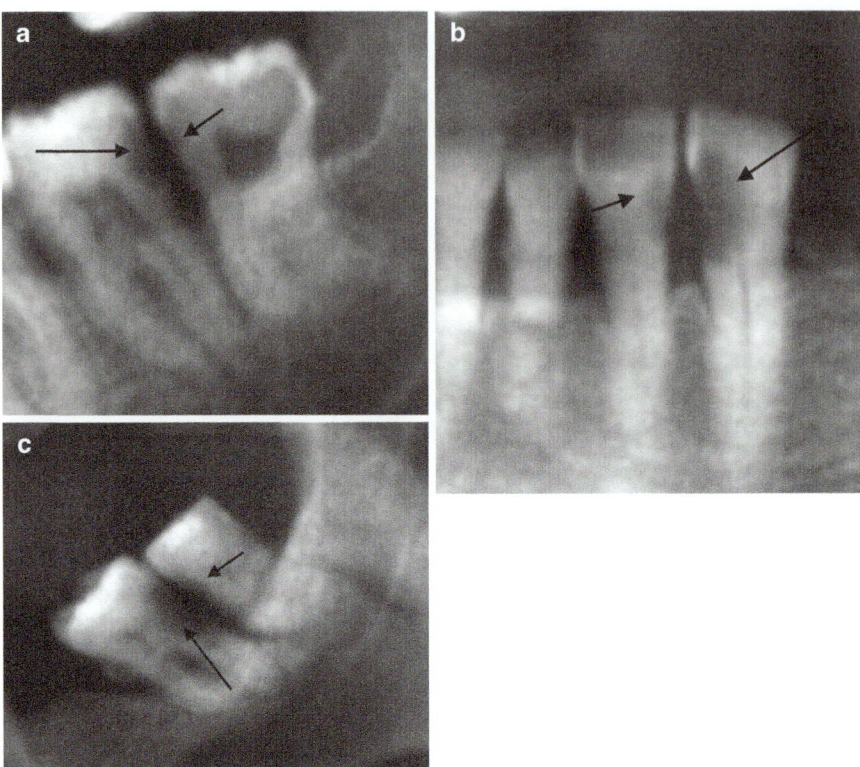

Fig. 4.7 Interproximal caries both in the medial side and distal side. (**a**) Distal caries (indicated by *short arrow*) affecting only the enamel and distal caries (indicated by *long arrow*) also affecting the dentine. (**b**) Mesial caries (indicated by *long arrow*) also affecting the pulp chamber and distal caries (indicated by *short arrow*) affecting only the dentine. (**c**) Distal caries (indicated by *long arrow*) affecting the pulp chamber and mesial caries (indicated by *short arrow*) limited to the dentine

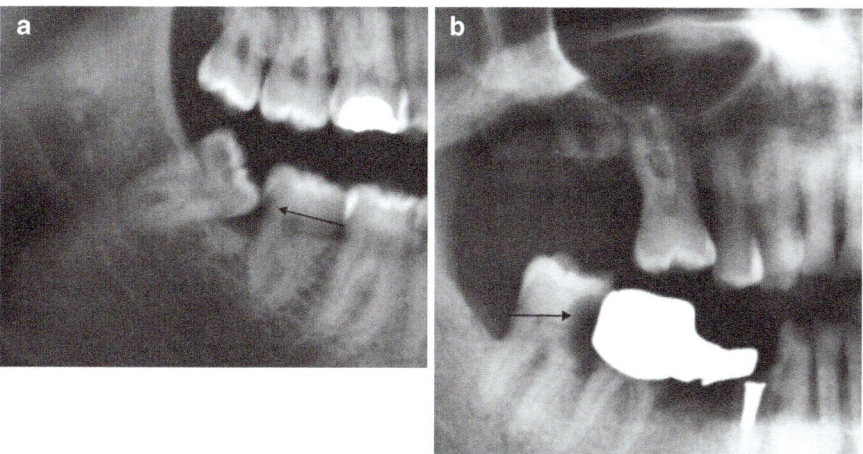

Fig. 4.8 (**a**) Distal interproximal caries (indicated by *arrow*) of 4.7 due to the impact with 4.8 in mesiodistal angulation, presenting occlusal caries. (**b**) Mesial interproximal caries of 4.7 (indicated by *arrow*) with overhanging crown capsule of 4.6

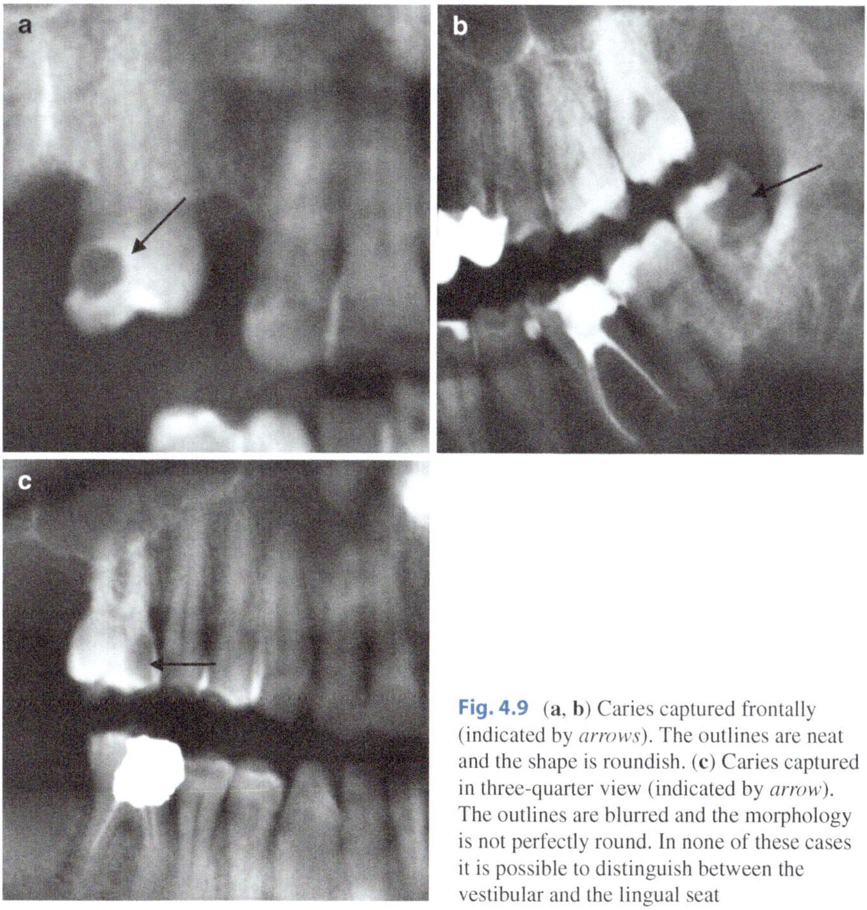

Fig. 4.9 (**a**, **b**) Caries captured frontally (indicated by *arrows*). The outlines are neat and the shape is roundish. (**c**) Caries captured in three-quarter view (indicated by *arrow*). The outlines are blurred and the morphology is not perfectly round. In none of these cases it is possible to distinguish between the vestibular and the lingual seat

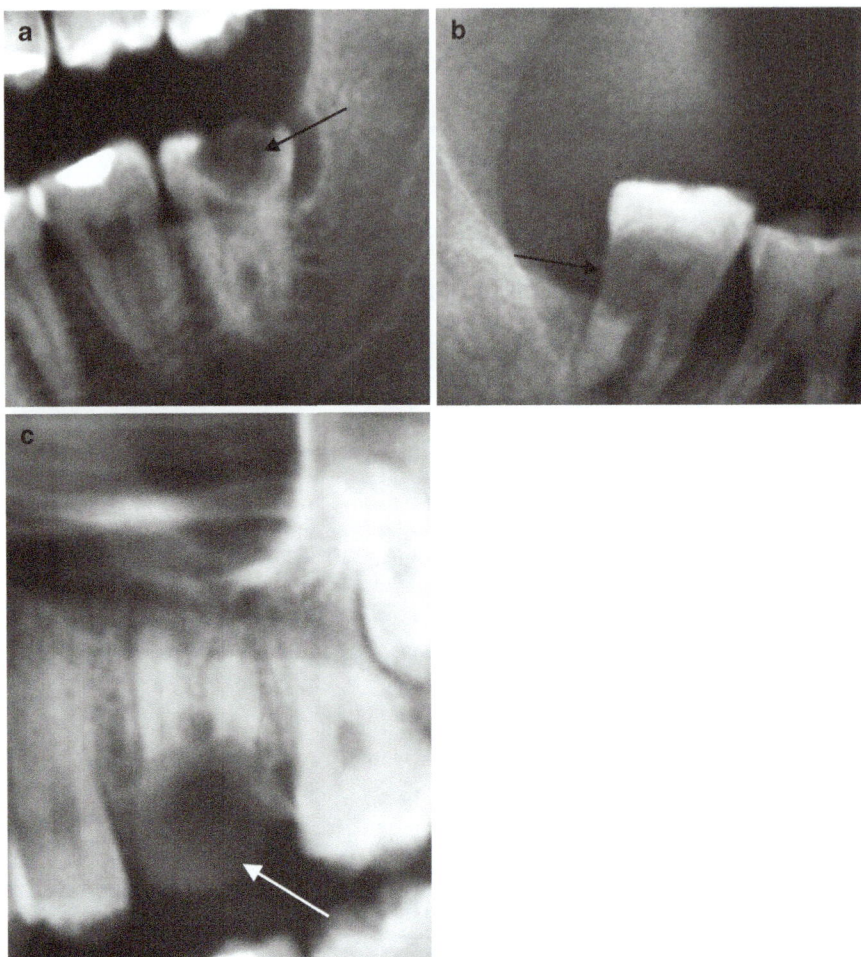

Fig. 4.10 (**a–c**) Wide carious lesions (indicated by *arrows*) in which the seat of origin cannot be traceable. (**b**) The affection of the radicular axis lines and therefore of the cementum. (**c**) The complete destruction of the crown

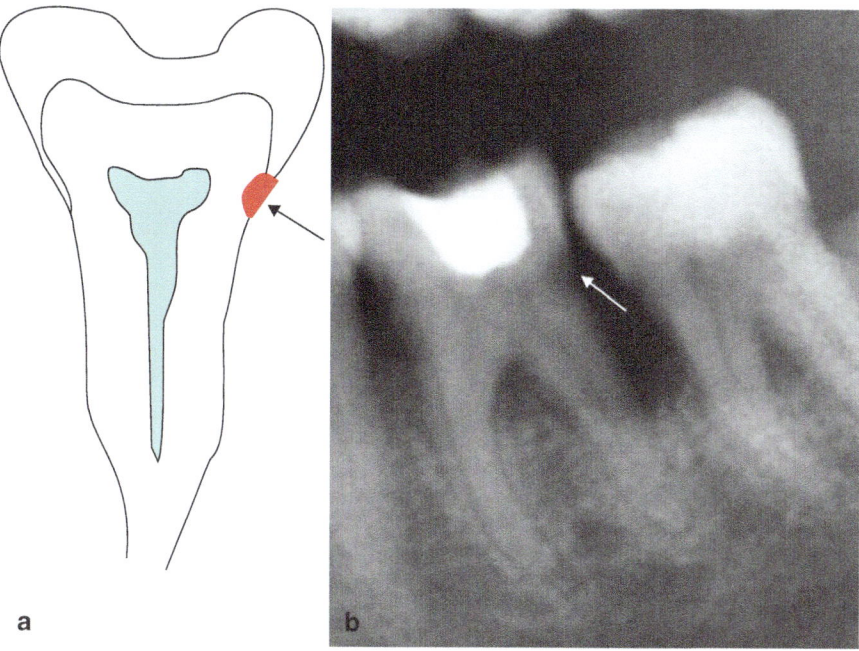

Fig. 4.11 Schematic (**a**) and radiological (**b**) model of how a small caries of the cementoenamel junction (indicated by *arrow*) can affect the dentine early

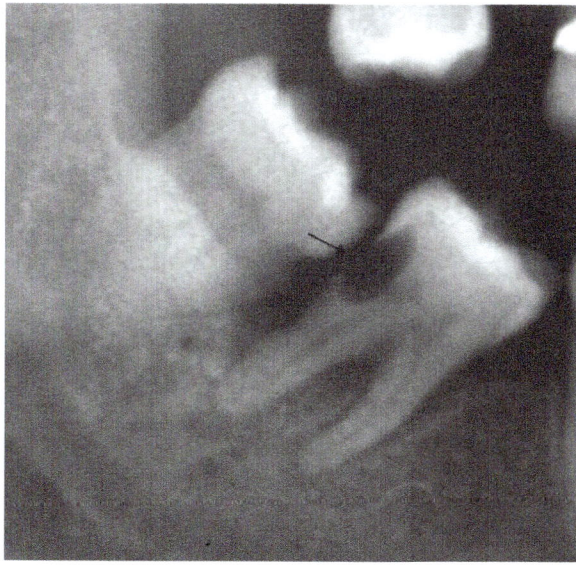

Fig. 4.12 Distal interproximal caries of the 4.7 with pit aspect. The gateway to the cavity is very narrow (it is indicated by *arrow*), while the cavity itself, however, extends deeply into the dentine

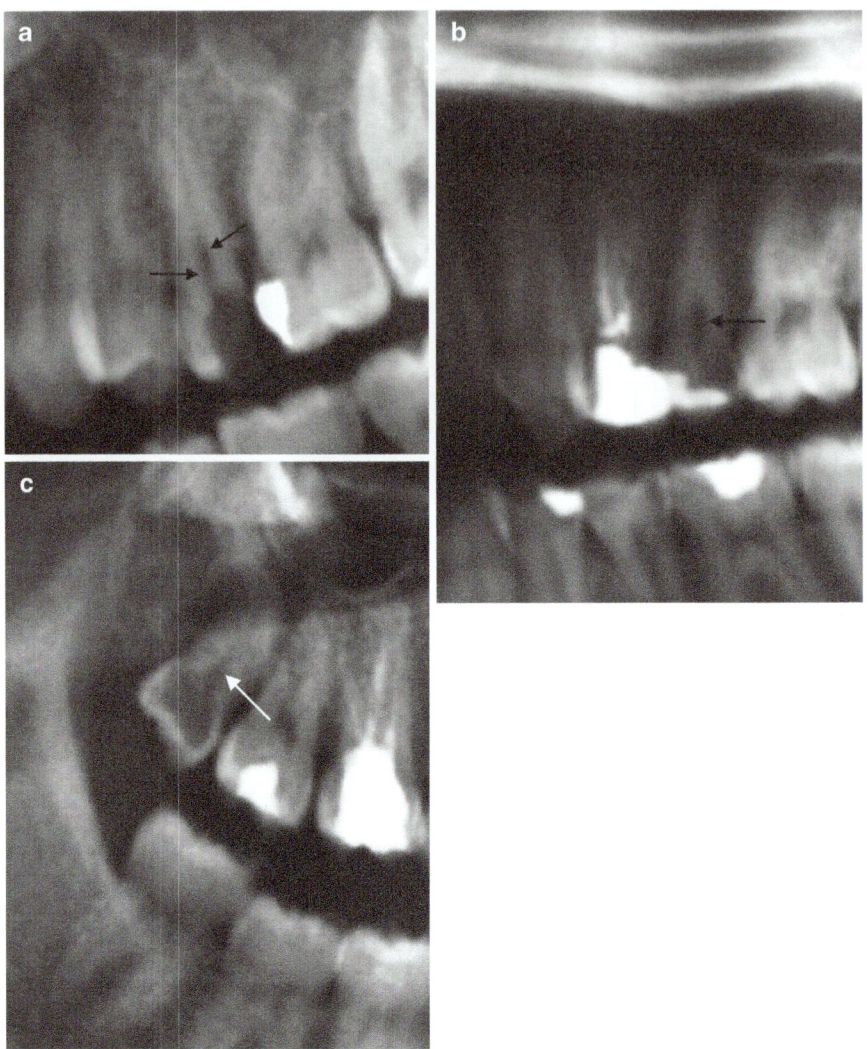

Fig. 4.13 (**a–c**) Caries associated to endodontic erosion phenomena of the pulp canal (it is indicated by *arrows*)

Fig. 4.14 Filled caries with likely obliteration of the pulp canal of the mesial root (indicated by *long arrow*). Good visibility of the pulp canal of the distal root (indicated by *short arrow*)

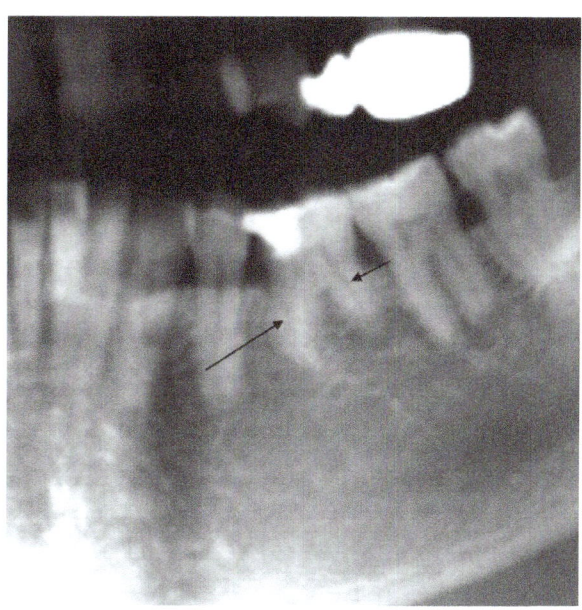

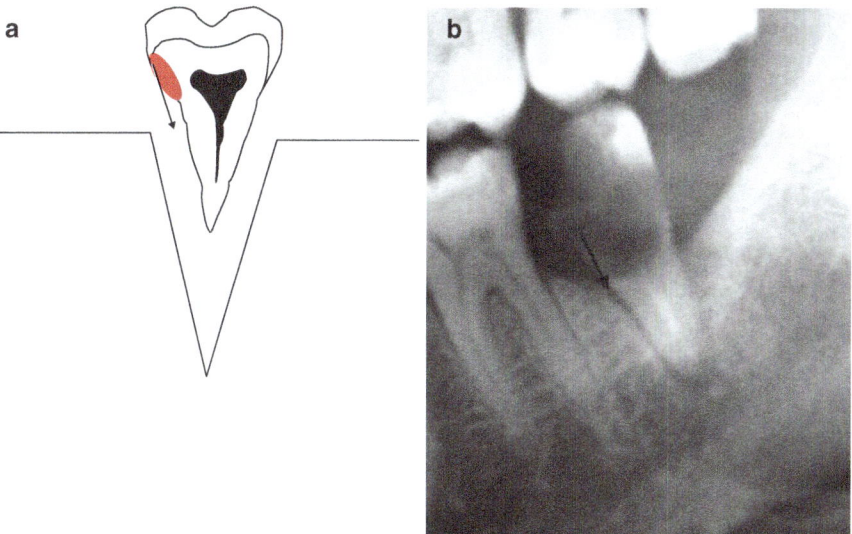

Fig. 4.15 Schematic diagram (**a**) and radiological representation (**b**) of the aggression of the periodontal space in the presence of caries (*arrow*)

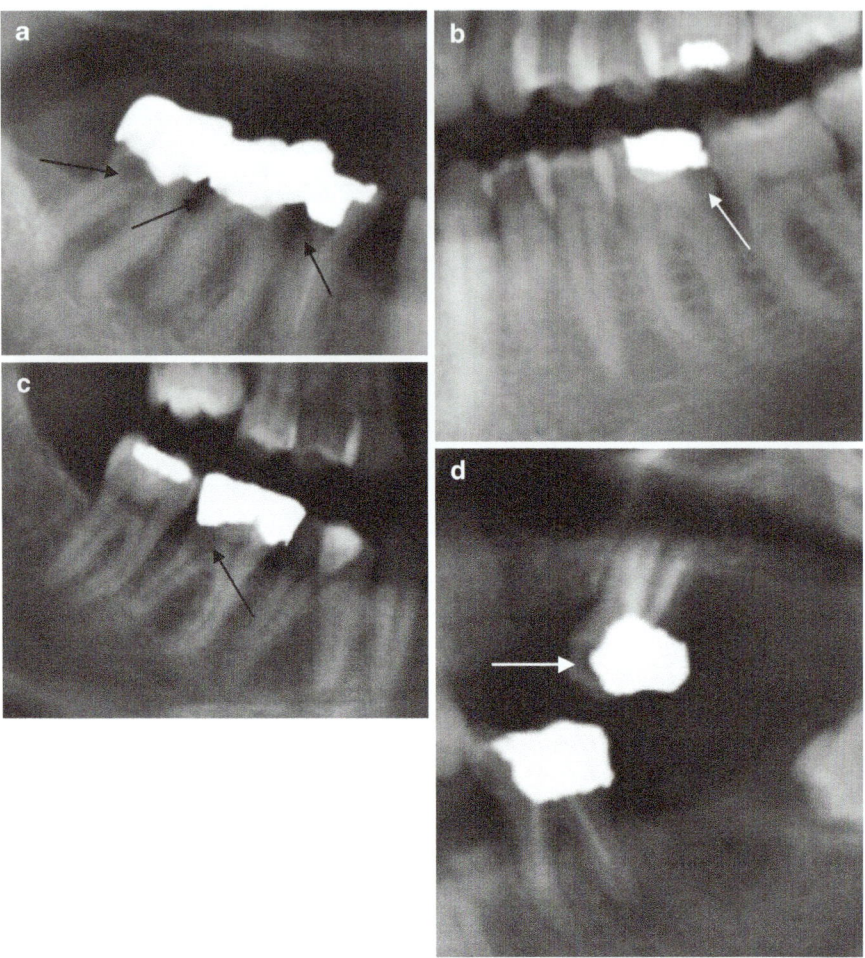

Fig. 4.16 (**a–d**) Different typologies of secondary caries (indicated by *arrows*)

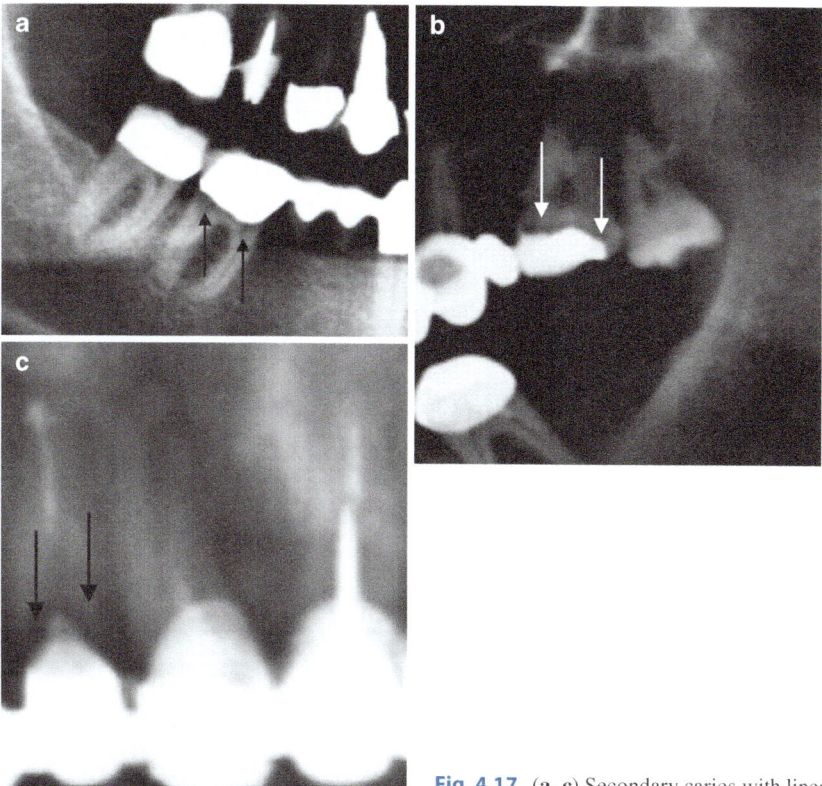

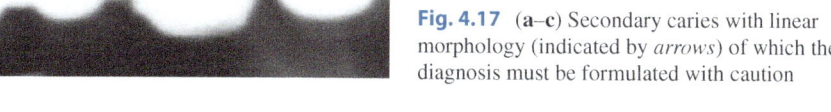

Fig. 4.17 (**a**–**c**) Secondary caries with linear morphology (indicated by *arrows*) of which the diagnosis must be formulated with caution

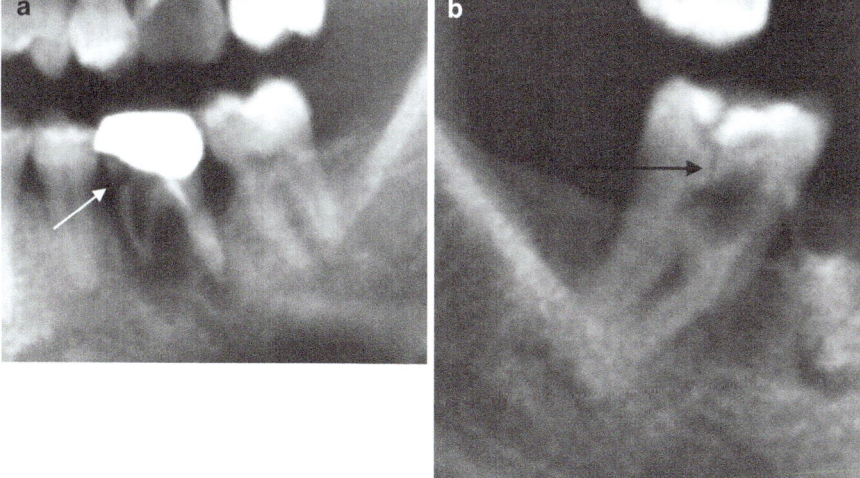

Fig. 4.18 Various types of dental fractures. (**a**) Fracture (indicated by *arrow*) associated to a serious endodontic damage with a consequent widening of the mesial root's radicular canal. (**b**) Occlusal caries with a thin line of crown fracture (indicated by *arrow*)

Fig. 4.19 False image of the edge of the cementoenamel junction's carious erosion (indicated by *arrow*)

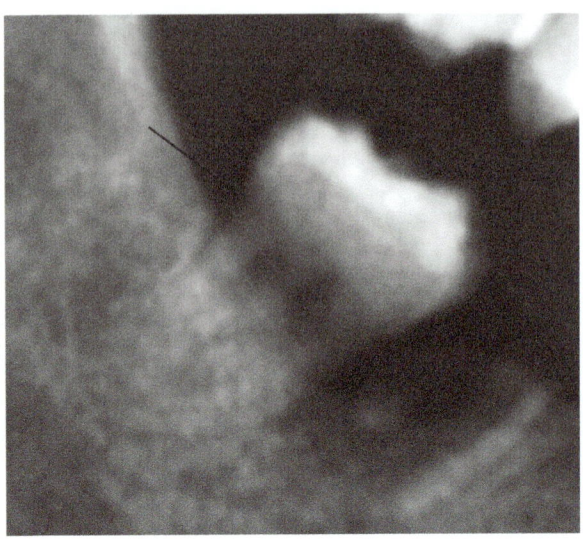

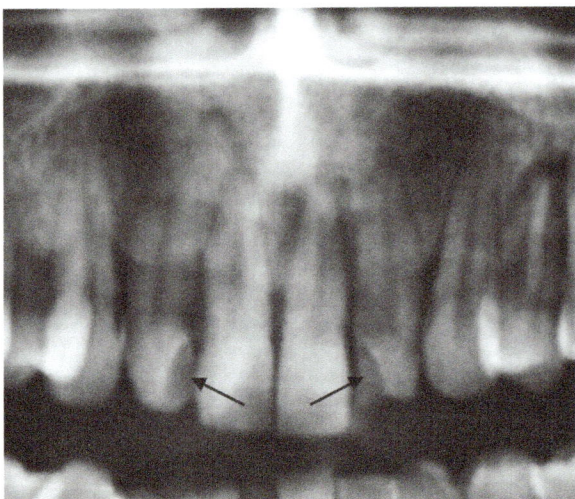

Fig. 4.20 False caries of the lateral incisors (indicated by *arrows*) due to dental repair procedure with radiolucent material

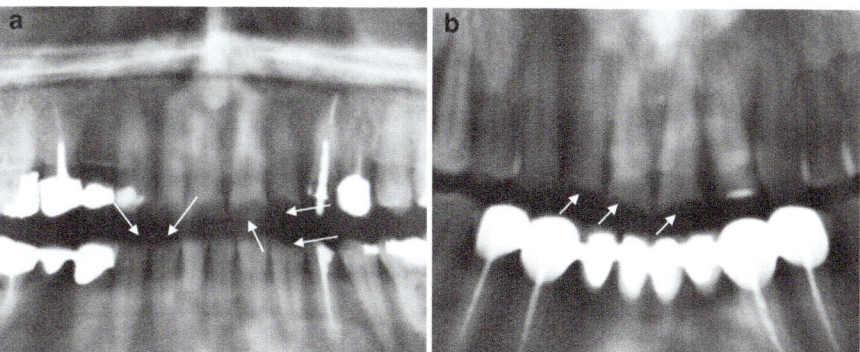

Fig. 4.21 (**a, b**) Two cases of abrasion of the frontal teeth's masticatory surface (indicated by *arrows*)

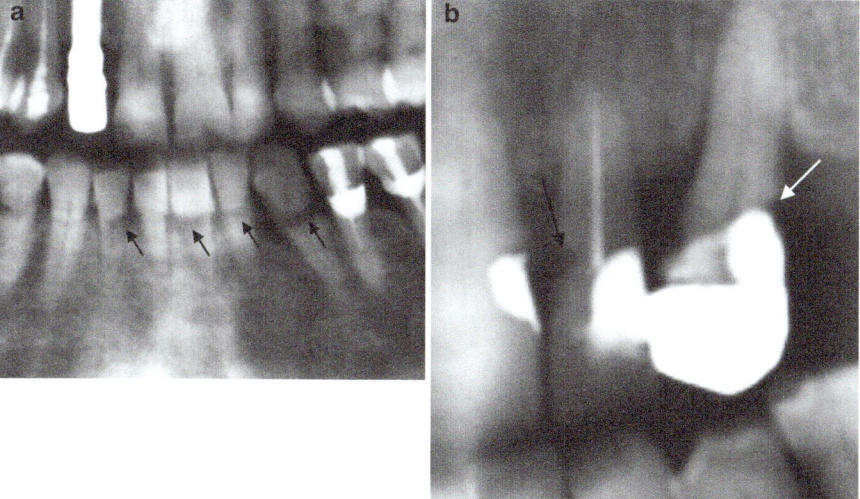

Fig. 4.22 (**a**) Linear fissure of the inferior incisors' neck and of 3.3 (indicated by *arrows*). (**b**) Triangular fissure (indicated by *arrows*)

Fig. 4.23 Triangular fissure with clear limits (indicated by *long arrow*) easily distinguishable by a real caries (indicated by *short arrow*)

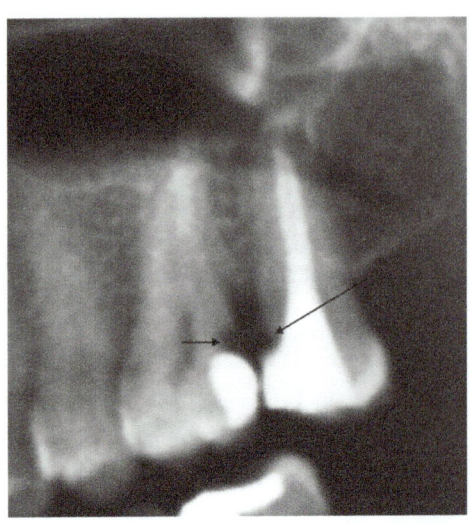

Suggested Reading

Akarslan ZZ (2009) Author's reply to the Letter to the Editor entitled "Gold standard for the comparison of the diagnostic accuracy of panoramic images for approximal caries detection" published in Dentomaxillofacial Radiology (2009;38:245). Dentomaxillofac Radiol 38(7):493

Akarslan ZZ, Akdevelio lu M, Güngör K, Erten H (2008) A comparison of the diagnostic accuracy of bitewing, periapical, unfiltered and filtered digital panoramic images for approximal caries detection in posterior teeth. Dentomaxillofac Radiol 37(8):458–463

Akkaya N, Kansu O, Kansu H, Cagirankaya LB, Arslan U (2006) Comparing the accuracy of panoramic and intraoral radiography in the diagnosis of proximal caries. Dentomaxillofac Radiol 35(3):170–174

Barr JH, Stephen RG (1980) Dental radiology. Saunders, Philadelphia

Bin-Shuwaish M, Dennison JB, Yaman P, Neiva G (2008) Estimation of clinical axial extension of class II caries lesions with ultraspeed and digital radiographs: an in-vivo study. Oper Dent 33(6):613–621

Cantelmi P, Singer SR, Tamari K (2010) Dental caries in an impacted mandibular second molar: using cone beam computed tomography to explain inconsistent clinical and radiographic findings. Quintessence Int 41(8):627–630

Clark HC, Curzon ME (2004) A prospective comparison between findings from a clinical examination and results of bitewing and panoramic radiographs for dental caries diagnosis in children. Eur J Paediatr Dent 5(4):203–209

Clifton TL, Tyndall DA, Ludlow JB (1998) Extraoral radiographic imaging of primary caries. Dentomaxillofac Radiol 27(4):193–198

Kamburoglu K, Kolsuz E, Murat S, Yüksel S, Ozen T (2012) Proximal caries detection accuracy using intraoral bitewing radiography, extraoral bitewing radiography and panoramic radiography. Dentomaxillofac Radiol 41(6):450–459

Ng MW, Chase I (2013) Early childhood caries: risk-based disease prevention and management. Dent Clin North Am 57(1):1–16

Pitts NB (1993) Current methods and criteria for caries diagnosis in Europe. J Dent Educ 57:409

Poyton HG (1980) Oral radiology. Williams & Wilkins, Baltimore

Thylstrup A, Fejerskov O (1996) Textbook of clinical cariology. Munkgaard, Copenaghen

Wenzel A (2009) Gold standard for the comparison of the diagnostic accuracy of panoramic images for approximal caries detection. Dentomaxillofac Radiol 38(4):245

White SC, Pharoah MJ (2000) Oral radiology: principles and interpretation. Mosby, St Louis

Periapical Lesions

5

Inflammatory **periapical lesions** turn out to be complex and can be confusing in some aspects, also for the experts. This is mainly due to the lack of pathognomonic radiological images, able to characterise the different pathological entities, and the lack of clinical verification which often characterises the OPT radiological reports.

Indeed, there is no doubt that the possibility of having clinical functional information at disposal (**sensitivity tests**, anamnestic confirmation, etc.) can be the key factor in precisely marking out the radiological images, which often are nonspecific.

On the basis of what is mentioned above, it is evident that, in the (very frequent) case of the evaluation of the radiological images in a context lacking of clinical information, the radiologist has to describe the picture accurately, without employing terms which subtend complex pathological realities (e.g. **apical granuloma**, acute **periapical abscess**), but describing only elementary alterations (**interruption of the lamina dura**, **periapical lytic lesion**, **perialveolar osteosclerosis**, etc.).

Nosography of Inflammatory Periapical Lesions

As explained above, even if in the majority of cases, the radiological image is to be considered as nonspecific, a brief nosologic overview of the topic seems to be useful (also in order to use a correct terminology).

Alterations of the periapical tissues can be triggered by inflammatory phenomena of endodontic or periodontal origin (Figs. 5.1a, b and 5.2a, b).

In the first case, the infectious process reaches the periapical region following alterations in the dental pulp, which in turn are caused by penetrating caries or by conditions which cause the contamination of the endodontic content (incongruous treatments, traumatic lesions, etc.)

Conversely, in the second eventuality, the periapical lesion derives from an infection of the periodontal space which represents a predetermined pathway of diffusion (this topic will be treated more extensively in the following chapter).

I. Pandolfo, S. Mazziotti, *Orthopantomography*,
DOI 10.1007/978-88-470-5289-5_5, © Springer-Verlag Italia 2013

From the clinical point of view, periapical alterations can be classified as acute, subacute and chronic.

Acute alterations are a consequence of oedematous or necrotic pulpitis, which in most cases, will not give rise to any radiologically recognisable modification.

Conversely, if the pathological process goes further forward, acute periapical abscess originates.

This last, if correctly and promptly treated, can evolve towards healing. Otherwise it can be characterised by a torpid and prolonged course (**subacute periapical abscess** and **chronic periapical abscess**). In this case it is followed by possible complications (fistulisation, osteomyelitis, apicolysis, etc.).

Further evolution of the lesion will gradually lead to its progression, with extended destructive phenomena of the alveolar cancellous bone (**chronic alveolitis**). These may or may not be associated to reactive sclerosis of the surrounding bone trabeculae (**osteitis condensans**).

Chronic lesions also include the apical granuloma.

This is a lytic lesion of granulomatous nature. Most of the time it is bacterially sterile and it has a scarce clinical appearance (it is often an asymptomatic lesion). However, it is also the expression of an infectious process of endodontic origin.

The presence of epithelial rests (**rests of Malassez**) in the context of granuloma can influence the cystic evolution, with the consequent formation of a radicular cyst (an entity which will be treated in Chap. 7).

Periapical Abscess

As previously explained, radiological images turn out to be generally nonspecific.

Conversely, the elementary alterations supporting them present a precise pathological significance.

It follows that the medical report will describe those alterations, avoiding the labelling of the lesions with terms which often turn to be imprecise, and even erroneous.

For this reason, the frequent impossibility of discerning a small chronic periapical abscess from an apical granuloma seems to be paradigmatic. This occurs if the morphological element is considered exclusively without any reference to clinical context.

Acute periapical abscess, if not treated by therapy, can appear as a minimal widening of the periapical periodontal space, which, in its early phases, can still be associated to the integrity of the lamina dura (Fig. 5.3a, b).

It seems to be evident that in such cases, the abscess diagnosis is not justified only on the basis of radiological alteration, as analogue modifications of the periodontal space can be supported by inflammatory phenomena. These are constituted only by oedema and cellular infiltrates which are not in purulent evolution.

Further progression of the lytic lesion of the periapical cancellous bone, along with the disappearance of the lamina dura, will create a clear abscessual collection.

In such a phase, the lesion will be characterised by blurred outlines because of the indistinguishable interface between the abscessual collection and the surrounding trabecular bone (Fig. 5.4a, b).

From one hand, the subsequent modifications of periapical abscess depend on the efficiency and the timeliness of therapeutic approach (both medical and odontoiatric); from the other hand, they depend on the patient's immune system capacity.

Indeed, the lesion, in those cases with a slightly aggressive course, will present a thin sclerotic delimitation representing a restraining reaction produced by the adjacent cancellous bone.

In such cases, as will be discussed later, the lesion will turn out to be indistinguishable from the apical granuloma (Fig. 5.5).

Abscesses with major aggresiveness and/or prolonged progression could sometimes be associated with more extended phenomena of osteosclerosis.

This last consideration is extremely indicative of the abscessual nature of the periapical lesion, which obviously has a chronic course (Fig. 5.6).

In those cases in which the resistance capacities of the host bone are not able to contain the further evolution of the morbid process, progressive growth of the abscessual collection occurs. The latter can sometimes reach conspicuous dimensions (Fig. 5.7a–c).

Fistulisation phenomena and massive destruction of the alveolar bone (chronic alveolar abscess) are included within the abscess' unfavourable evolution.

Fistulisation of the periapical abscess can spread along various pathways depending on the localisation (superior vs. inferior maxillary) and on its prevalent seat (vestibular or lingual) (Fig. 5.8a, b).

This can occur for the erosion of the cortical bone in the vestibular or lingual side. In such cases, the phenomenon is not visible through OPT for the already mentioned impossibility of its tridimensional representation (as is well known, such type of fistula is well-documented through computed tomography).

Conversely, OPT can provide documentary evidence of the fistulous paths originating with respect to the mandibular canal or to one of its alveolar branches. This is due to the fact that, in such cases, the fistulous path is generally oriented according to the frontal plane (Fig. 5.9a–c).

A more arduous task is the evaluation of possible fistulisation and/or involvement of the maxillary sinus by periapical lesions situated on the superior arcade.

Indeed, in such cases, the evaluation of the state of cortical bone, which marks off the maxillary sinus, is difficult and even insidious, if only using OPT.

This evaluation turns out to be possible only when the cortical interface between the maxillary sinus and the periapical lesion is represented tangentially by the incident beam.

Therefore, it becomes radiographically recognisable (Fig. 5.10a, b).

Conversely, in the majority of cases, the evaluation is beyond OPT possibilities. This is due to the extreme thinness of the aforementioned cortical bone along with its innumerable variations of orientation and unfavourable contrast conditions (Fig. 5.11a–c).

It must be added that OPT is a technique scarcely efficient to give evidence of slight inflammatory thickening of the sinus mucosa.

It must also be considered that the endosinusal area is also protected by the periosteal membrane, covering the internal wall (**Schneider's membrane**). It is obviously radiolucent, therefore not radiographically detectable.

In short, in the evaluation of the relations between a periapical lesion and the maxillary sinus, computed tomography is much more effective than OPT.

Regarding the chronic alveolar abscess, it represents the extreme evolution of the morbid process, in a destructive sense. This causes extended substance losses of the cancellous bone which is adjacent to the alveolus (Fig. 5.12a–c).

In the presence of this last entity, due to the complete disintegration of the normal alveolar architecture, it is impossible to distinguish if the process has endodontic or periodontal origins.

However, it must be said that such distinction has only an academic meaning as it lacks any practical use.

Apical Granuloma

Apical granuloma represents the other face of chronic inflammatory lesions of the periapical region. From the pathological point of view, it is constituted by an accumulation of sterile, inflammatory granulation tissue. It is characterised by a slow increase at the expenses of the surrounding spongious bone.

On the clinical point of view, the apical granuloma turns out to be oligo- or asymptomatic, and at times it represents just an occasional finding.

Radiologically the only differential element with respect to the chronic abscess is represented by the sharpness of the outlines which are often detected by a thin sclerotic line (Fig. 5.13a–c).

It is clear that such a morphological element is quite unpredictable as the chronic abscess can often show the same characteristics of the apical granuloma. Conversely, the latter can be characterised by blurred outlines, in relation to possible septic reactivation (which can characterise the natural course of the apical granuloma).

Briefly, differential diagnosis between the two entities is not possible in the majority of cases, if effectuated through radiographical examination only.

The presence of fistulisation phenomena, generally absent in the apical granuloma, is more oriented to a diagnosis of chronic abscess.

The possible presence of epithelial rests (**rests of Malassez**) in the tissue structure of the apical granuloma can cause, following the cystic evolution of the rests, the transformation of the granuloma into radicular cyst.

Even though the two entities are completely different from the pathological point of view (see Chap. 7), radiological differential diagnosis between a big apical granuloma and a small radicular cyst in evolution is not possible.

For reasons of descriptive and semantic nature, in order to distinguish the two entities, the dimensional criterion is usually considered. Its limit of about 12–15 mm of diameter represents the transition between a granuloma in cystic evolution and a clear radicular cyst (Fig. 5.14a–c).

Pararadicular Inflammatory Lesions

A particular aspect of the inflammatory lesions is represented by the pararadicular localisation.

This peculiar manifestation is related to the externalisation of the flogistic endodontic process which spreads along the lateral dental canals, rather than through the main radicular canal.

In literature, such lesions are called **pararadicular granulomas**.

The definition turns out to be inaccurate as the differential problem between granulomas and chronic abscesses exists also for the aforementioned localisations.

Similarly to the periapical lesions, the distinction can be made only by the finding of a thin sclerotic hem which itself, however, is far from specific (Fig. 5.15a–d).

Phenomena of reactive radicular hypercementosis (to be distinguished from idiopathic hypercementosis, originating for unknown reasons in a normal dental element) are included among the phenomena linked to the presence of an inflammatory lesion with chronic course (Fig. 5.16a, b).

Destructive alterations of the apex and/or radicular axis (**rhizolysis and pathological apicolysis**) are also considered as a possible complication of chronic inflammatory lesions (Fig. 5.17a–d).

Finally, there are also cases in which the apical-radicular destruction is followed by phenomena of **radicular remodelling** (Fig. 5.18).

Periapical and Periradicular Sclerosing Lesions

To conclude the dissertation of periapical and periradicular lesions, osteosclerotic alterations, which can occur in the aforementioned seats, must be mentioned separately.

Literature concerning this topic often shows the possibility for apical granulomas and/or chronic periapical abscesses which evolve into resolution (both spontaneous and after conservative treatment), to turn into osteosclerotic lesions.

Such an assertation, even if based on incontrovertible observations, must take into account the existence of other entities which can give rise to similar and even identical situations which therefore are not always distinguishable.

Such field includes **cementoma** and **islands of compact bone**.

Cementoma is often erroneously included among the odontogenic neoplasms.

Conversely, it represents a lesion which is generically classified into the field of bone dysplasias of unknown origin (from which arises the denomination **cemento–osseous dysplasia** or **periapical cemental dysplasia**).

In its initial phase, cementoma appears as a lytic area of the periapical cancellous bone. Its outlines are sharp and it is not radiographically distinguishable from an apical granuloma, except for the fact that the tooth which is affected is normal in the other aspects.

In its further progression, the lesion, which is always clinically asymptomatic, is characterised by an evolution towards progressive osteosclerosis. In this intermediate phase, the lesion will turn out to be easily diagnosable (Fig. 5.19a, b).

Conversely, as a result of a further evolution towards sclerosis, the lesion transforms itself into an entirely calcified small mass which is characterised by high opacity and regular and clear outlines, strictly adherent to the apex region (Fig. 5.20a, b).

At this stage of its evolution, cementoma can be confused with a possible compact island (which is also an asymptomatic lesion without any clinical relevance) which accidentally projects itself in correspondence with the tooth's apical region.

To summarise, differential diagnosis of the entirely osteosclerotic periapical lesions is fundamental with the following considerations:

1. Cementoma always occurs in a healthy tooth and is not dissociable from the tooth apex and/or from the periodontal space because it originates from the cementum.
2. Granulomatous and/or abscessual lesion, evolved into osteosclerosis, occurs in a deeply altered tooth, and it generally shows quite irregular morphology.
3. Compact island (often multifocal) can project itself in correspondence with both a normal tooth and a pathological one. It is however well dissociable from the periodontal space and is always localised externally to it (Figs. 5.21a–c, 5.22a–c and 5.23).

Image Gallery

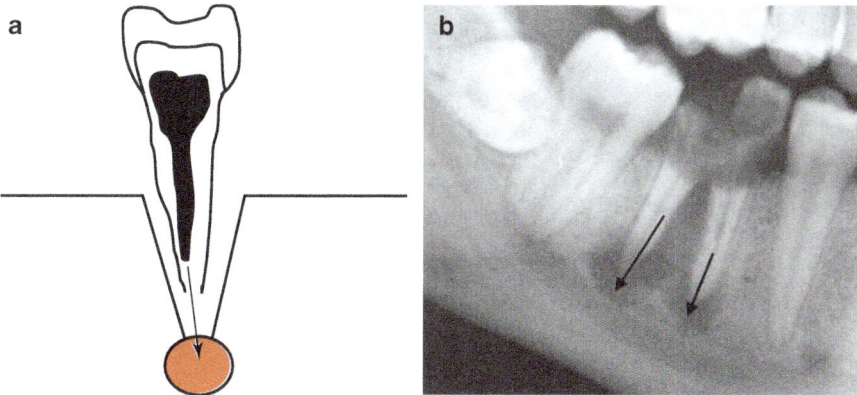

Fig. 5.1 Schematic diagram (**a**) and radiological representation (**b**) of periapical lesion of endodontic origin (*arrows*)

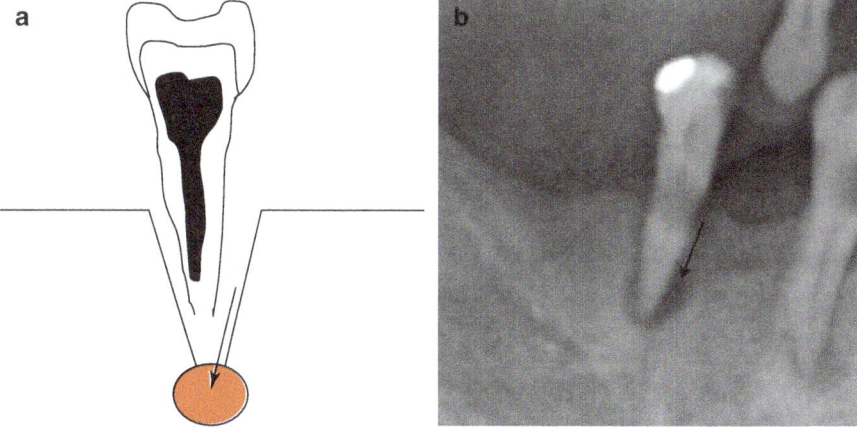

Fig. 5.2 Schematic diagram (**a**) and radiological representation (**b**) of periapical lesion of periodontal origin (*arrows*)

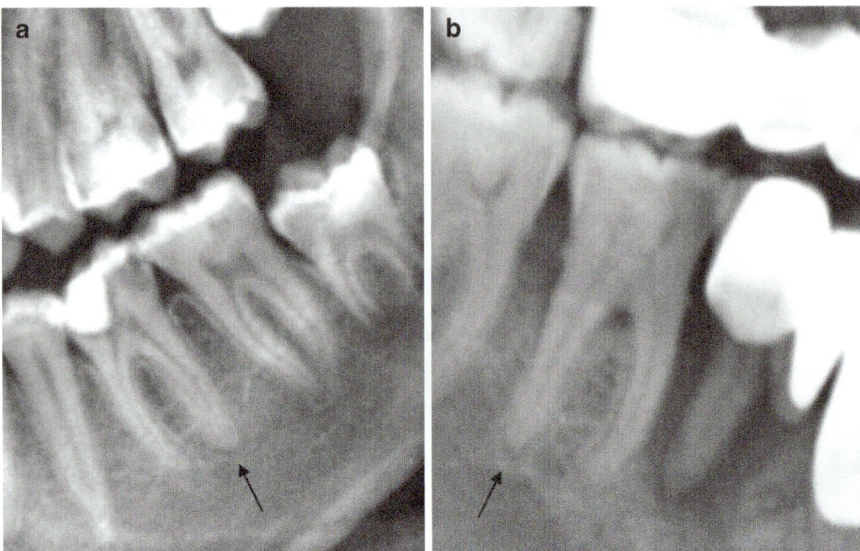

Fig. 5.3 Two cases of minimal and initial periapical inflammatory alteration (indicated by *arrows*). The periodontal space seems to be widened with integrity of the lamina dura. (**a**) Secondary caries of 3.7. (**b**) Caries of 4.6

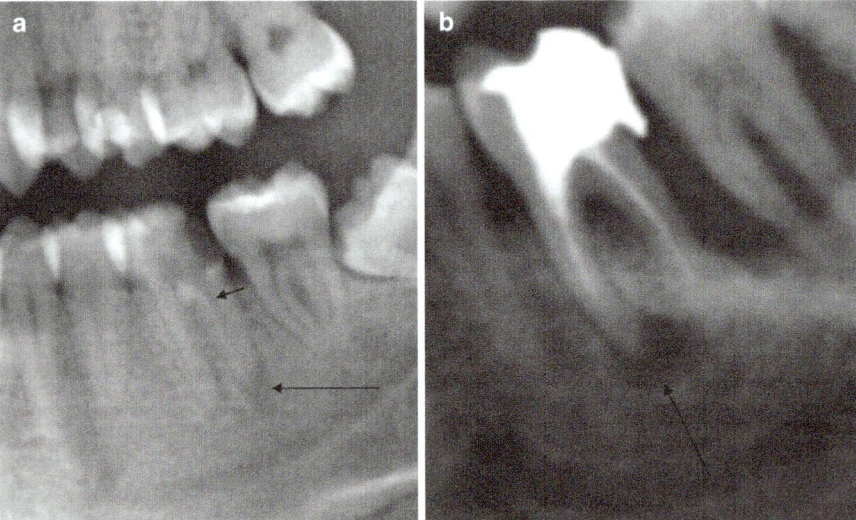

Fig. 5.4 Further progression of the periapical lesions (indicated by *arrows*) in abscessual direction, with interruption of the lamina dura. (**a**) Shows penetrating caries of 3.6 with widening of the canal due to endodontic damage (it is indicated by the *short arrow*). In picture (**b**) the lesion seems to be more extended and with blurred outlines

Fig. 5.5 Two periapical lesions (abscesses) in different evolutionary stages, but with phenomena of perifocal sclerosis (indicated by *arrows*). The lesions are indistinguishable from apical granuloma

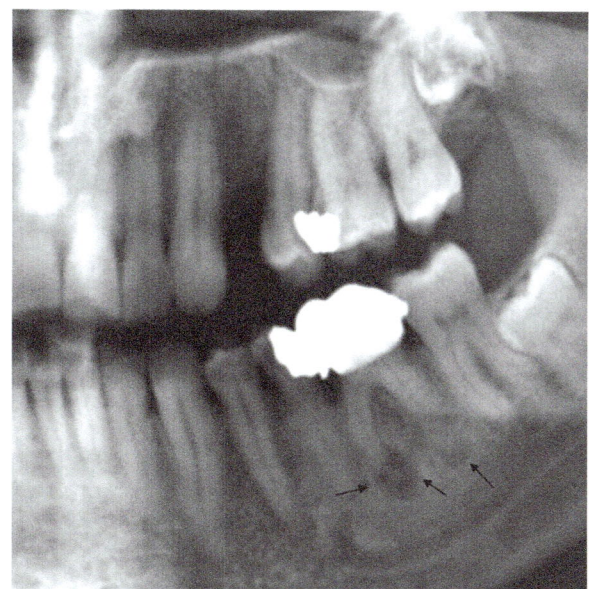

Fig. 5.6 Periapical lesion delimited by a thick vallum of sclerosis of the surrounding spongiosa (indicated by *arrows*). This element confirms the abscessual nature of the periapical lesion

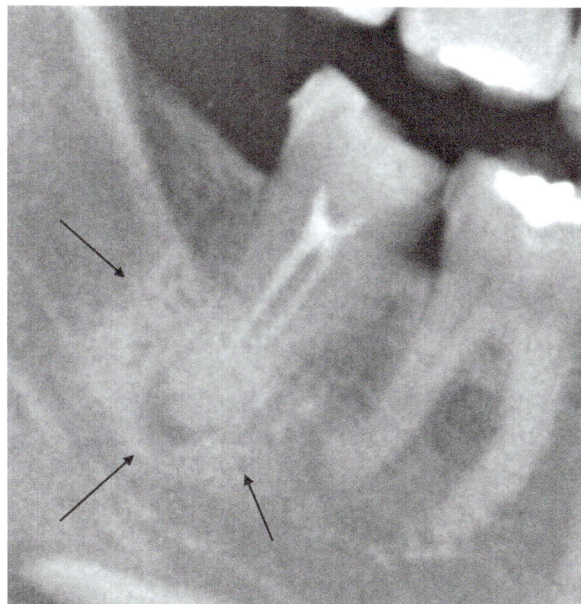

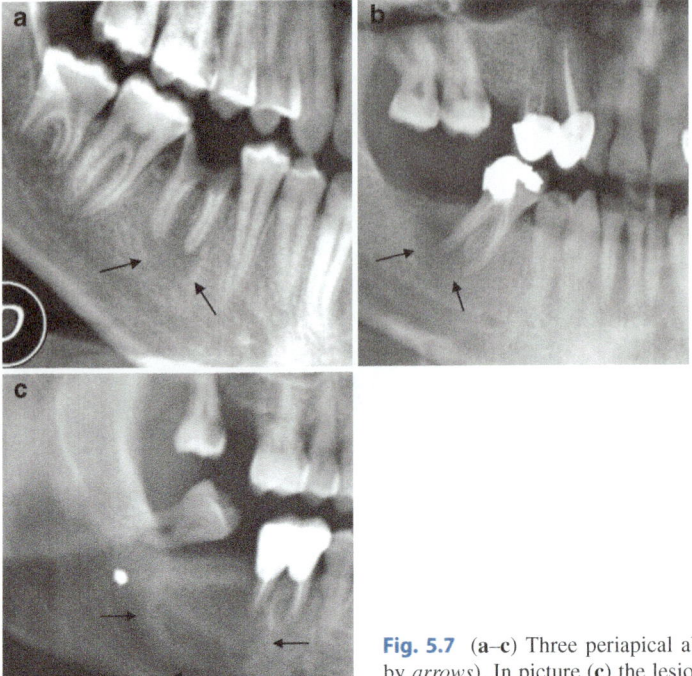

Fig. 5.7 (**a–c**) Three periapical abscesses (indicated by *arrows*). In picture (**c**) the lesion is delimited by a thin band of osteosclerotic reaction

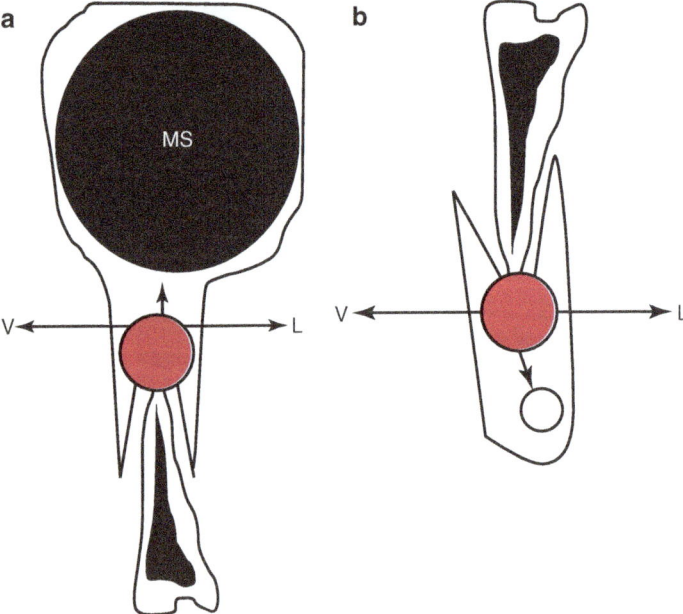

Fig. 5.8 Schematic diagram illustrating the fistulisation courses of the periapical abscess. (**a**) Frontal view of the superior maxillary. The *arrows* indicate the courses in vestibular (*v*) and lingual (*L*) seats and towards the maxillary sinus (*MS*). (**b**) Frontal view of the inferior maxillary with courses in vestibular (*v*) and lingual (*L*) seats and towards the mandibular canal

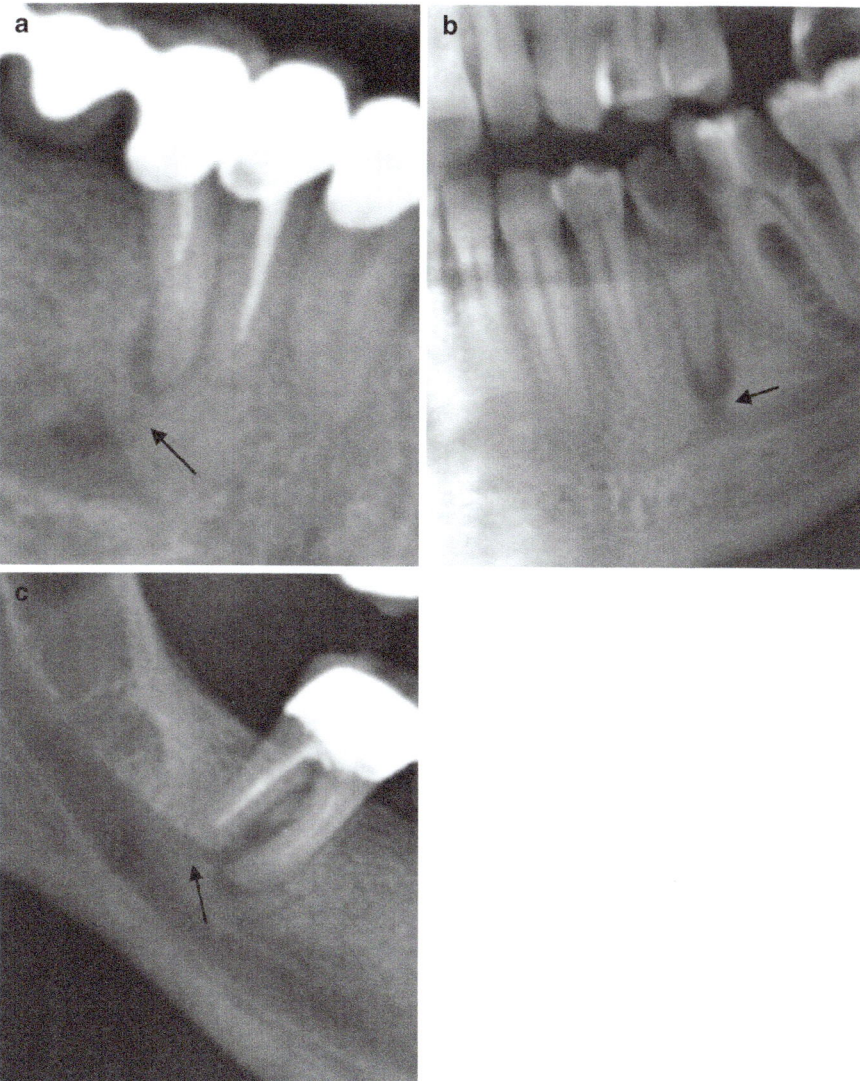

Fig. 5.9 (**a**, **b**) Periapical abscesses connected by fistulous paths (indicated by *arrows*) to the mandibular canal. In picture (**c**) the abscess is fistulised in an alveolar canaliculus which appears widened (indicated by *arrow*)

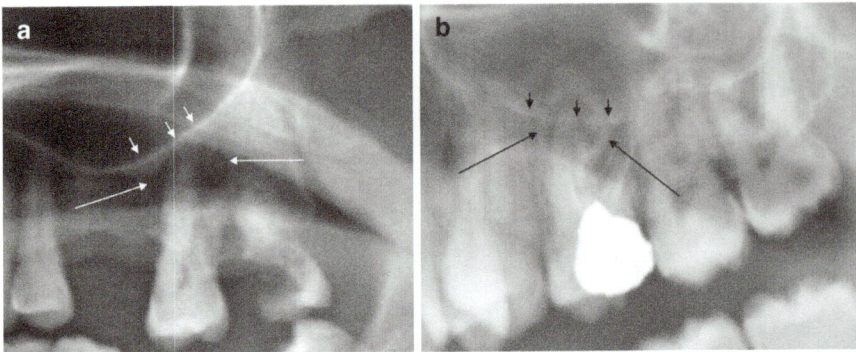

Fig. 5.10 (**a, b**) Periapical lesions (indicated by *long arrows*). The cortical (indicated by *short arrows*) which represents the floor of the maxillary sinus is detectable in both cases indicating the absence of fistulisation

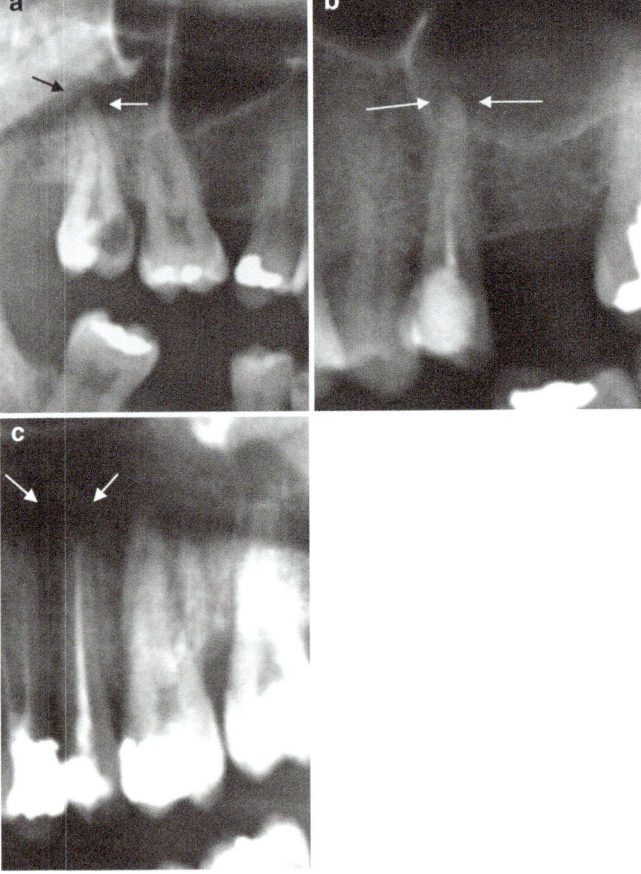

Fig. 5.11 (**a–c**) Periapical lesions (indicated by *arrows*) in relation to the maxillary sinus. A reliable evaluation of the state of the cortical bone, which marks off the maxillary sinus, is never possible

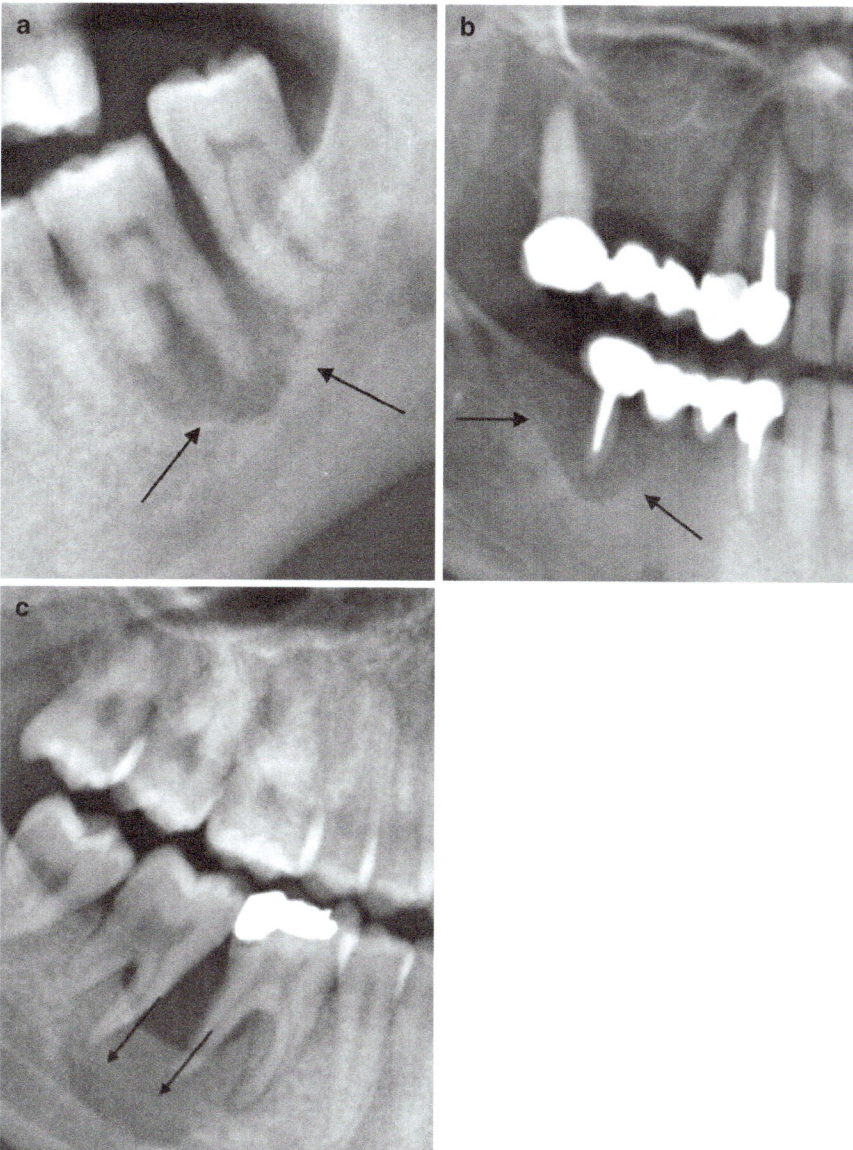

Fig. 5.12 Three cases of chronic alveolar abscess (indicated by *arrows*). (**a**) Resorption phenomena of the radicular axis. (**b**) A widely disintegrating perialveolar process. The tooth is characterized by an endodontic post. (**c**) The lesion causes the disintegration of the cortical of the mandibular canal (indicated by *arrows*)

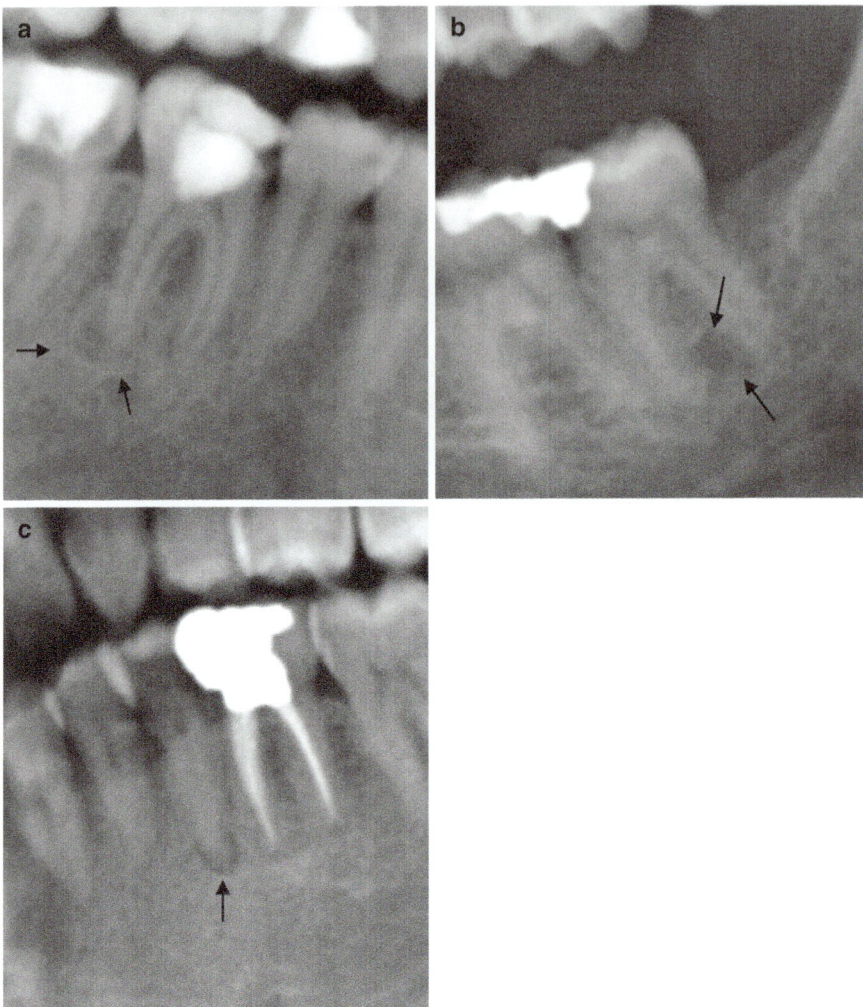

Fig. 5.13 (**a–c**) Periapical lesions (indicated by *arrows*) that, for the sharpness of their outlines and the thin sclerotic line, suggest the presence of apical granuloma

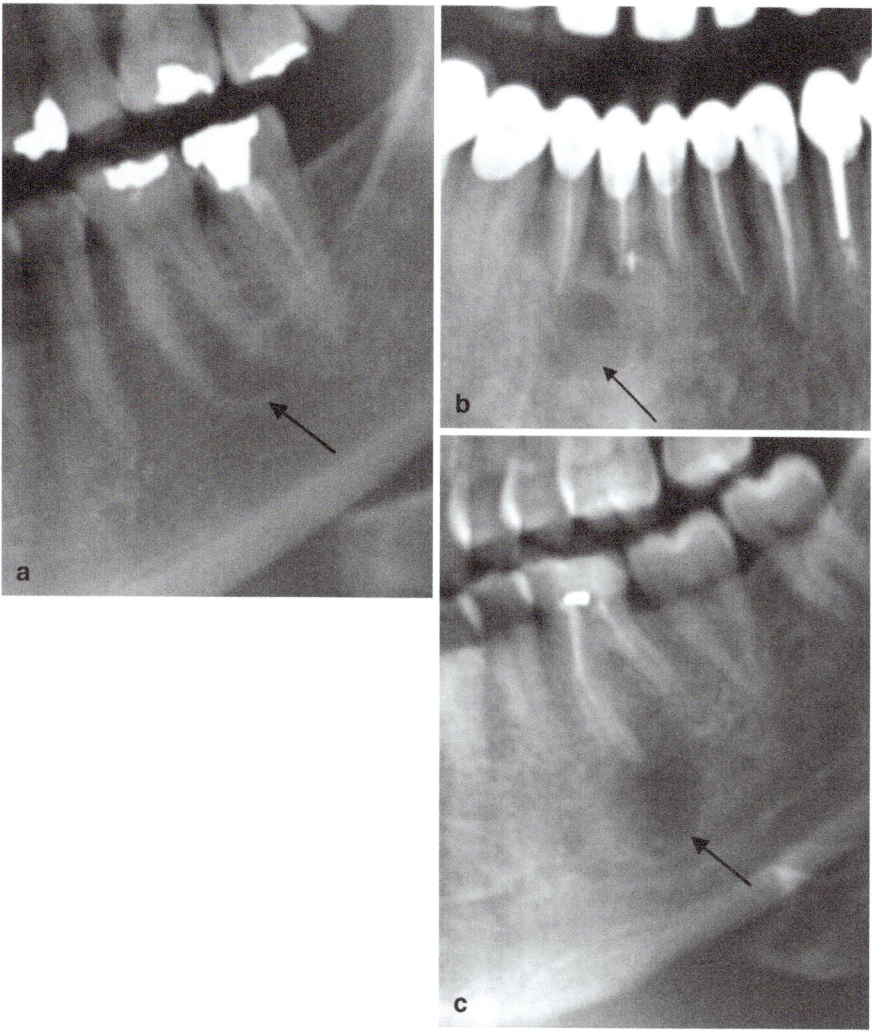

Fig. 5.14 (**a–c**) Three periapical lesions compatible with the diagnosis of apical granuloma in cystic evolution (*arrow*)

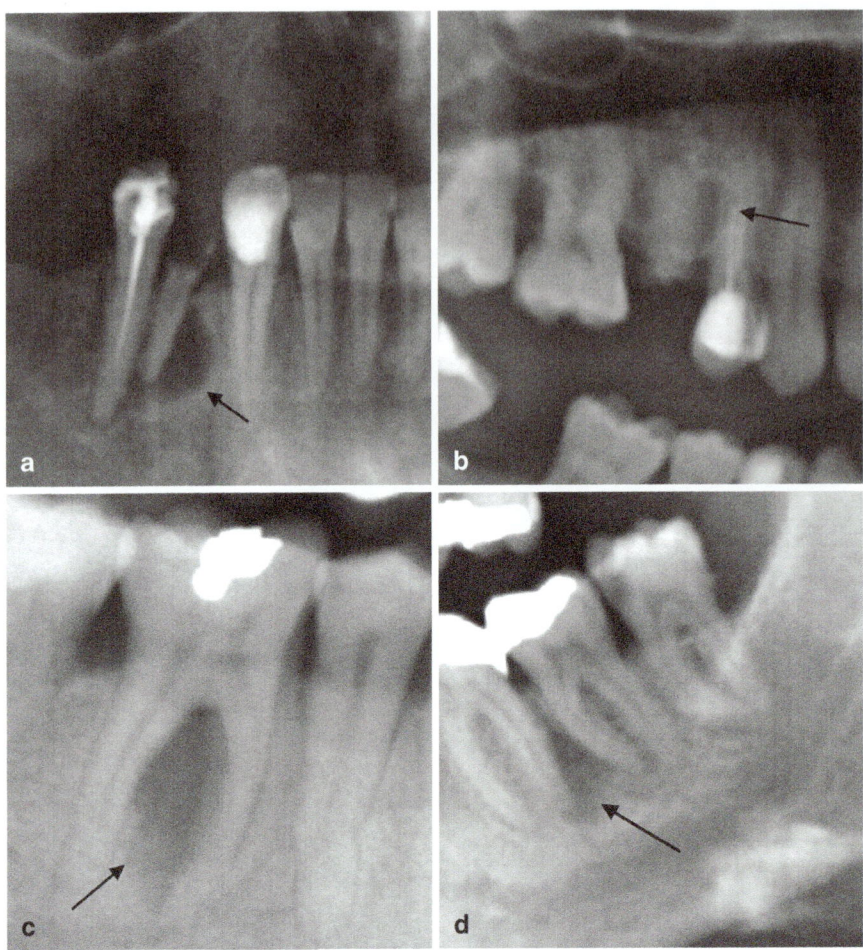

Fig. 5.15 (**a–d**) Periradicular lesions (indicated by *arrows*). (**a, b**) Lesions delimited by sclerotic hem. (**c, d**) Lesions showing blurred outlines

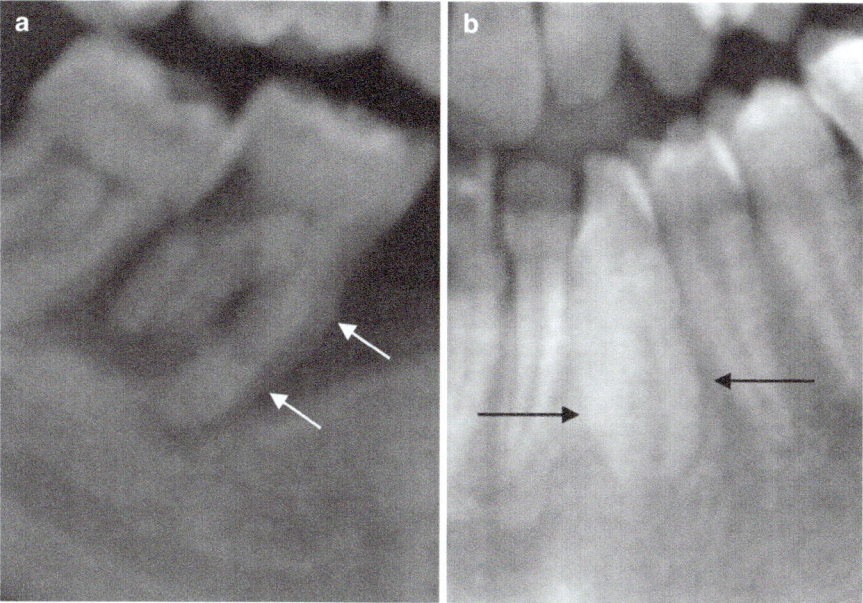

Fig. 5.16 (**a**) Reactive hypercementosis (indicated by *arrows*). (**b**) Idiopathic hypercementosis (indicated by *arrows*) in the element which is normal in the other aspects

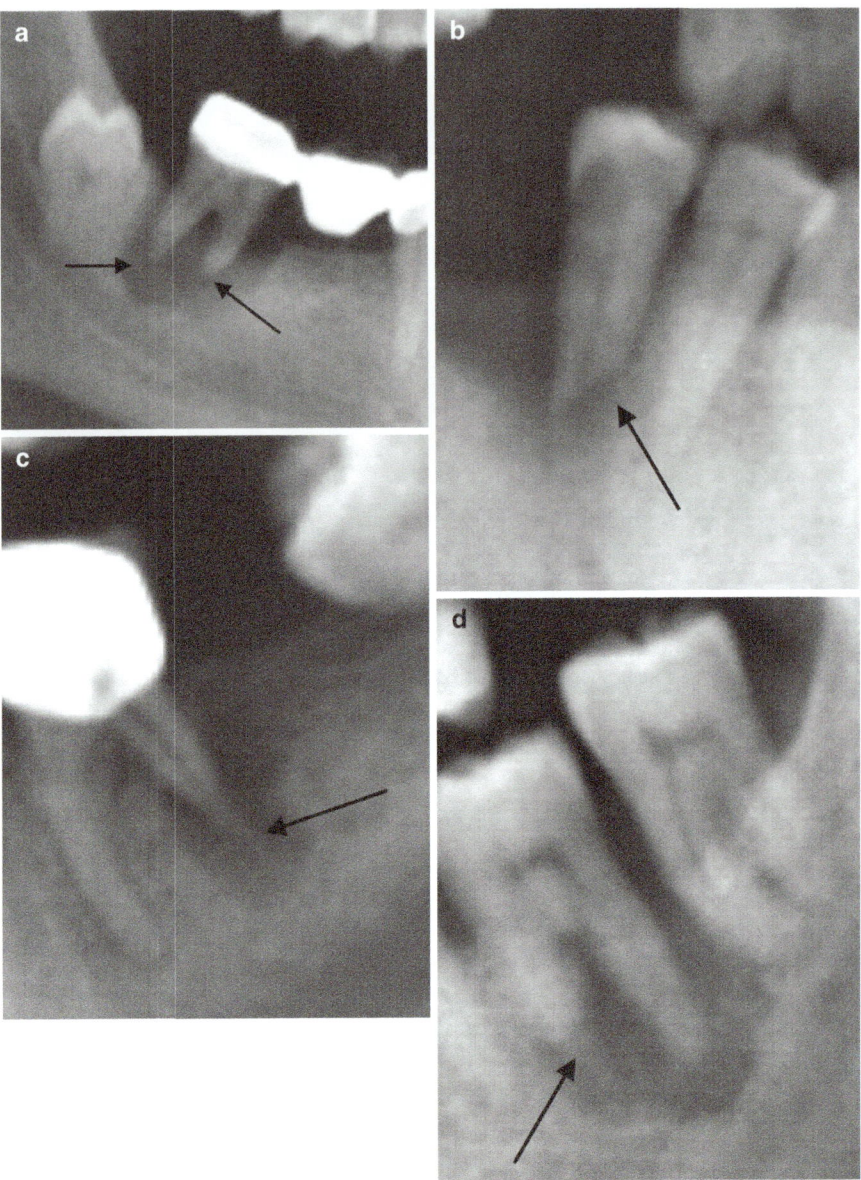

Fig. 5.17 (**a–d**) Different typologies of apico-rhizolysis (indicated by *arrows*) in periapical radicular lesions

Fig. 5.18 Phenomena of **radicular remodelling** (indicated by *arrows*)

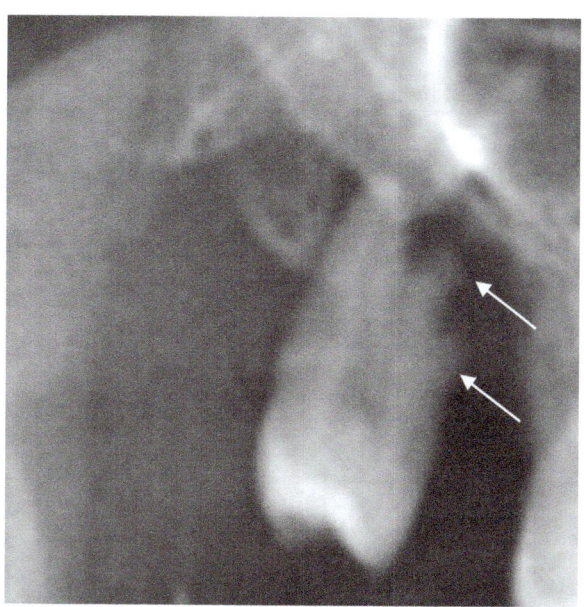

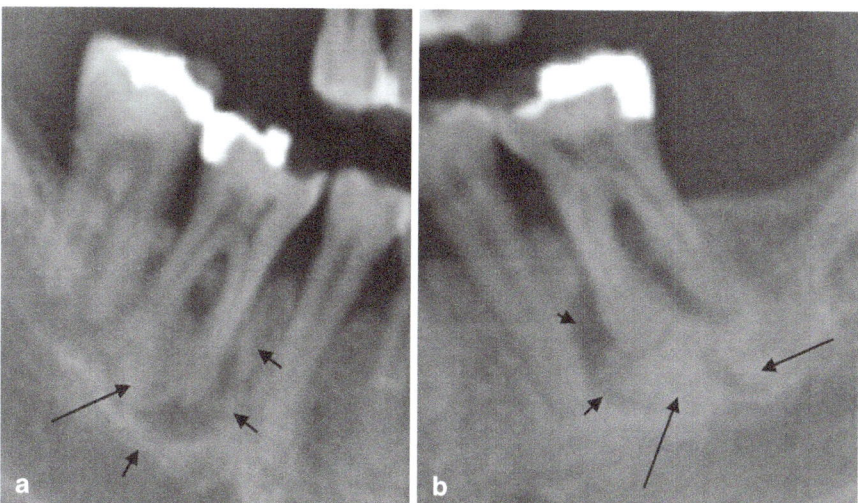

Fig. 5.19 (**a**, **b**) Two cases of cementoma in intermediate evolution. Presence of the lytic component with clear outlines (represented by *short arrows*) and of the osteosclerotic component (indicated by *long arrows*)

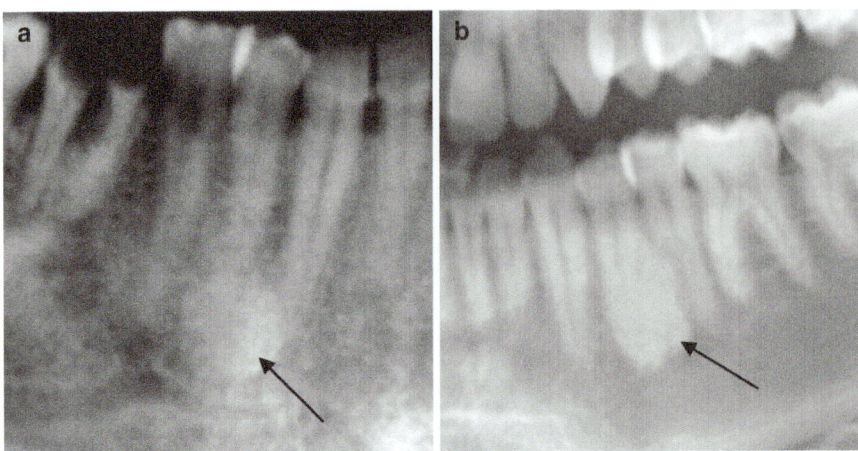

Fig. 5.20 (**a, b**) Two cementomas in complete osteosclerotic evolution (indicated by *arrows*)

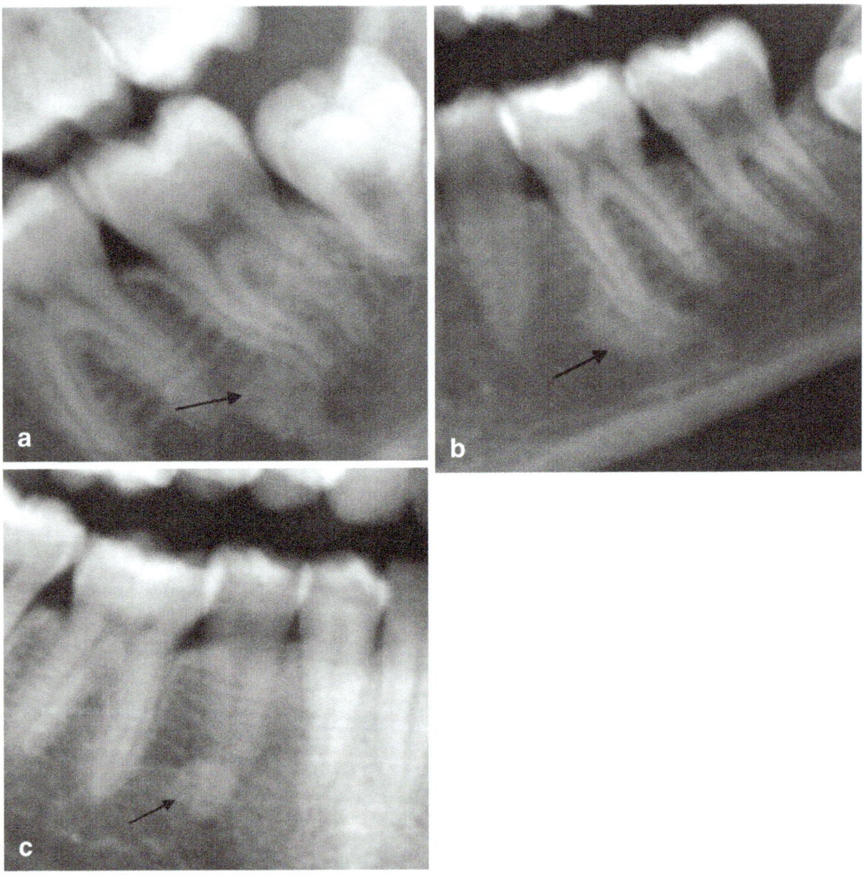

Fig. 5.21 (**a–c**) Three cases of compact island (indicated by *arrows*) in which opacity is dissociable from the apical region and the periodontal space

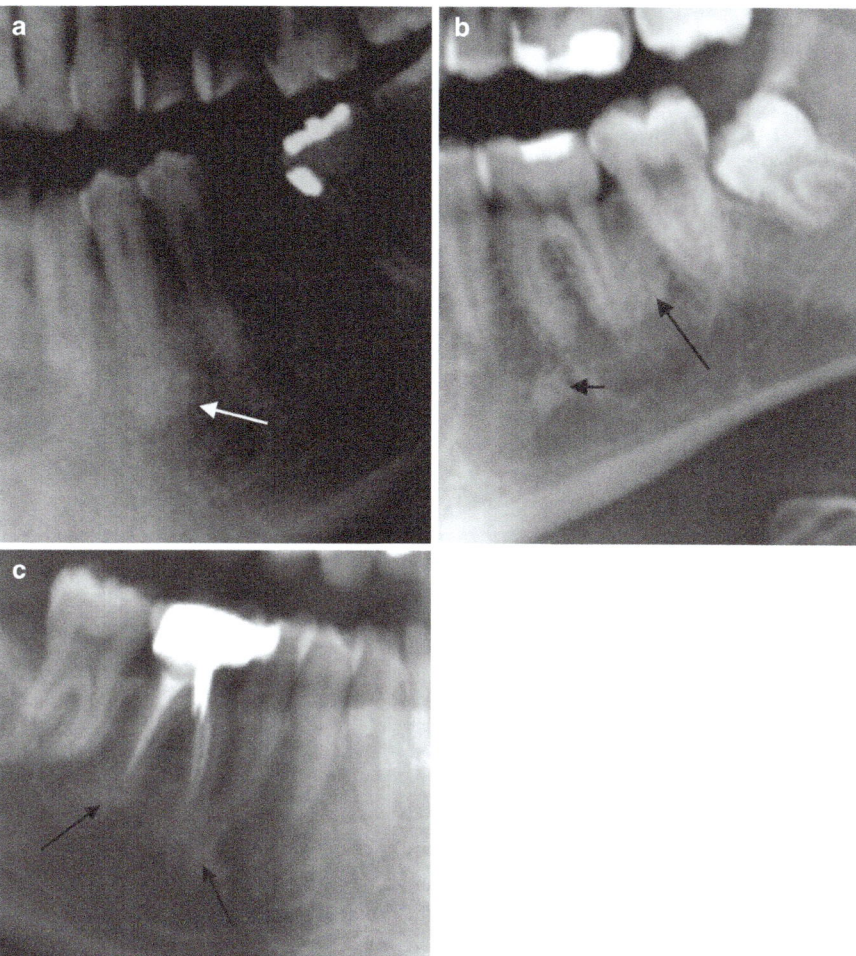

Fig. 5.22 (**a**) Periapical sclerotic lesion (indicated by *arrow*), not dissociable from the apex, in a healthy tooth, cementoma. (**b**) Periradicular sclerotic area, dissociable from the periodontal ligament (indicated by *long arrow*), with another further areola of sclerosis (indicated by *short arrow*), compact island. (**c**) Areas of periapical sclerosis with irregular outlines (indicated by *arrows*) in a tooth with endodontic treatment (evolution in sclerosis of flogistic periapical lesions)

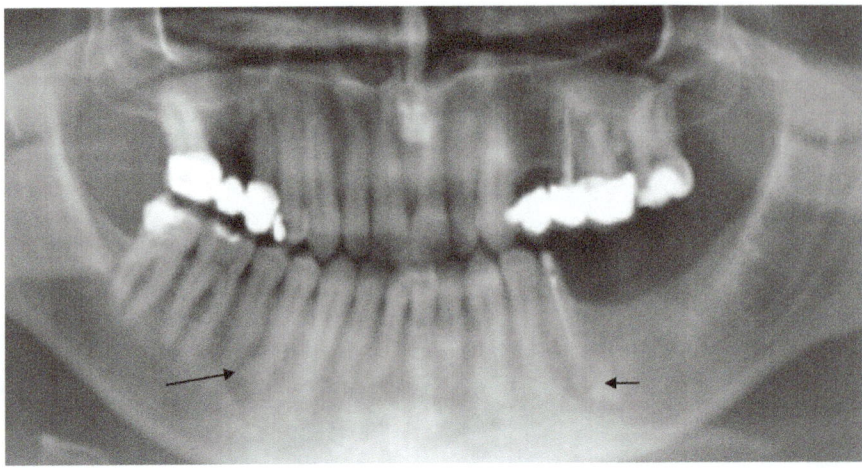

Fig. 5.23 *Long arrow*, area of periapical sclerosis in a normal tooth, cementoma. *Short arrow*, area of periapical sclerosis which is very irregular in a tooth with previous endodontic treatment (flogistic lesion evolved in sclerosis)

Suggested Reading

Alsufyani NA, Lam EW (2011) Cemento-osseous dysplasia of the jaw bones: key radiographic features. Dentomaxillofac Radiol 40(3):141–146

Barr JH, Stephen RG (1980) Dental radiology. Saunders, Philadelphia

Bergmans L, Van Cleynenbreugel J, Verken E et al (2002) Cervical external root resorption in vital teeth. J Clin Periodontol 29(6):580–585

Bulut EU, Acikgoz A, Ozan B, Zengin AZ, Gunhan O (2012) Expansive focal cemento-osseous dysplasia. J Contemp Dent Pract 13(1):115–118

Carrillo C, Penarrocha M, Ortega B, Martí E, Bagán JV, Vera F (2008) Correlation of radiographic size and the presence of radiopaque lamina with histological findings in 70 periapical lesions. J Oral Maxillofac Surg 66(8):1600–1605

Chadwick JW, Alsufyani NA, Lam EW (2011) Clinical and radiographic features of solitary and cemento-osseous dysplasia-associated simple bone cysts. Dentomaxillofac Radiol 40(4):230–235

Leach HA (2001) Radiographic diagnosis of root resorption in relation to orthodontics. Br Dent J 190(1):16–22

McNab S et al (2000) External apical root resorption following orthodontic treatment. Angle Orthod 70(3):227–232

Sameshima GT, Asgarifar KO (2001) Assessment of root resorption and root shape: periapical vs panoramic films. Angle Orthod 71(3):185–189

White SC, Pharoah MJ (2000) Oral radiology: principles and interpretation. Mosby, St Louis

The Periodontal Disease

6

Periodontopathies (or Parodontopathies) are affections of complex etiopatho-genesis. This is related to the often indissoluble link between a variably associated component of inflammatory origin and relevant dystrophic damage, with a greater or lesser extent.

This morbid process starts at the level of the gingival margin, and it extents itself progressively to the whole periodontal apparatus.

In its earlier stage the **periodontal disease** is characterised by the interruption of the **tooth-gingival connection** with retraction of gingiva towards the apical region. This alteration causes the uncovering of the cementoenamel junction and the pro-gressive destructive change of the supporting structures of the teeth (enlargement of the periodontal ligament space and resorption of the alveolar bone), with the forma-tion of pathological recesses between the gingiva, the alveolar bone and the tooth, known also as the **gingival and alveolar sockets**.

The most recent literature has clearly indicated and emphasised that the peri-odontal disease is multifactorial in its origin and is characterised by the coexistence between inflammatory and degenerative phenomena.

Therefore, on the basis of what is mentioned above, the terms of **paradentosis** or **pyorrhoea** turn out to be descriptively obsolete as they are mainly related to the dystrophic aspects rather than the inflammatory ones.

For the same reason, the more generic term of periodontopathy seems to be pref-erable to periodontitis (and indeed widely employed in literature and in clinical practice), as the latter seems to emphasise more the inflammatory aspects than the dystrophic ones, which are always present in practice.

The most recent findings on this topic include the following clinical-anatomic entities in the field of the periodontopathies:

- Chronic periodontopathy (or periodontitis)
- Aggressive periodontopathy (or periodontitis)
- Ulcero-necrotic periodontopathy (or periodontitis)

Chronic Periodontopathy (or Periodontitis)

This is the most common pathological entity which is typically more frequent in adults.

Clinical signs are represented by gingival inflammation, bleeding that is spontaneous or caused by instrumental manoeuvres, loss of the gingival connection and retraction followed by the resorption of the alveolar bone, with the consequent formation of gingival and alveolar sockets.

In the early stage the disease can show itself with **gingivitis** and appears slowly progressive. It can exacerbate when immune defences are reduced.

Pathological effects accumulate in the course of life until adult age is reached, when the destructive effects of the disease are evident. The degree of this destruction depends on plaque levels, smoke habit, stress, possible diabetes and efficiency of the immune system.

Smokers show an increased risk (three to seven times more likely) of contracting chronic periodontal disease compared to the general population.

In these subjects, prognosis is less favourable as the smoke can attenuate inflammation, hiding the real extent of the pathology.

Aggressive Periodontopathy or Periodontitis

It comprises rare forms characterised by rapid progression. It generally appears during puberty (**juvenile periodontitis**), often in localized form. Generalized form is obviously more serious and mainly hits young adults, but also older patients even if both forms (localized or generalized) are supported by a genetic predisposition. The infection from *Actinobacillus actinomicetecomitans* seems to be more involved in the focal variety, while *Porphyromonas gingivalis* and *Bacteroides forsythus* play a significant role in the generalised form.

In young patients, the diagnosis of aggressive periodontitis is based on the finding of rapid bone destruction and loss of connection, along with a disproportion between bacterial deposits and degree of periodontal destruction, in patients without relevant systemic diseases.

Ulcero-necrotic Periodontopathy or Periodontitis

Ulcero-necrotic periodontitis is a rare destructive event in the periodontal apparatus, characterised by gingival margins and papillae which are ulcerated and necrotic. These are covered by a pseudomembranous material. It is prevalent in youths (20–25 years old) in Third World countries.

Necrotic lesions develop rapidly and painfully, often with spontaneous bleeding.

Gingival necrosis, which affects interdental papillae, spreads itself into the alveolar bone, causing its destruction. Lymphadenopathy, fever and general malaise can appear in association with such pathology. Oral hygiene is typically very poor; this is due to a lack of dental brushing, as subjects find it particularly painful.

The disease does not seem to stem from the action of a precise microbial strain. However, it is now believed that it has multifactorial origin, in which the effects related to the metabolic products of the bacterial plaque coexist with those belonging to systemic diseases (AIDS, leukaemia, measles, chickenpox, tuberculosis), malnutrition, smoke, stress, depression, scanty oral hygiene, etc.

There is no doubt that, in the diagnostic evaluation and in the estimation of the damage caused by the periodontal disease, the roles of clinical observation and anamnestic analysis turn out to be significant. Conversely, the task of diagnostic imaging in general, and of OPT in particular, seems to be ancillary to the clinical diagnosis. This is due to the fact that such techniques are restricted to a descriptive and qualitative analysis of the elementary alterations which give rise to the various pathological scenarios.

In other words, radiological reports should not include expressions such as the following: 'acute periodontitis', 'chronic periodontitis' or other conjectures of differential diagnosis which are not part of OPT diagnostic possibilities.

The use of obsolete terms such as 'pyorrhoea' or 'paradentosis' should be avoided. As an alternative, terms like 'periodontopathy' or 'periodontal alteration' could be employed. They are quite generic appellations, but sufficiently indicative of the pathological alterations taken into exam.

Elementary Alterations of the Periodontium

As the prime mover of most periodontopathies is represented by **gingivitis**, which is not radiologically evaluable, the analysis of the periodontium's elementary alterations will be fundamentally focused on the following entities:
1. Tartar deposits
2. Resorption of the alveolar bone and of the alveolar sockets
3. Secondary alterations of the radicular apparatus

Tartar Deposits

Tartar deposit, as widely known, plays a significant role on the cascade of events which cause the onset of periodontal disease.

Indeed, gingival retraction, in association with poor oral hygiene, creates a biological environment capable of facilitating the stagnation and the deposit of calcareous material. Once such material has assumed a spicular morphology, which can be exuberant to a greater or lesser extent, it causes further gingival damage due to its mechanical action.

Therefore, typical morphology of tartar deposits is represented by the spicular apposition which can develop both above and under the gingiva.

It is extremely clear that **deposits below the gingival margin** are difficult to be visually evaluated. Moreover, these need to be radiologically detected, as they are characterised by a major pathological relevance.

Tartar deposits can be found both in patients with minimal and initial periodontal alterations and in the presence of serious anatomical-radiological situations (Figs. 6.1 and 6.2).

Spicula usually originates at the level of the cementoenamel junction but can, rarely, be localised more distally, in the adjacent radicular surface (Fig. 6.3).

In addition to the typical spicular morphology, tartar deposit can appear, even if only rarely, with various morphological aspects (Figs. 6.4 and 6.5).

Resorption of the Alveolar Bone (Horizontal or Vertical/Angular)

In the natural course of periodontal disease, the first alterations, which occur at the level of the alveolar bone component, are represented by the phenomena of demineralisation and resorption of cortical and cancellous bone. These are an effect of the chemical inflammation agents.

It is known that quantitative evaluations (thickness measurements) and qualitative evaluations (attribution of the skeleton structure to a certain category) are tasks pertaining to CT.

Therefore, OPT turns out to be mainly limited to the morphological judgement of these alterations.

The aforementioned alterations can vary in grade from minimal to serious, the latter of which is characterised by depletion of the alveolar bone.

From a general point of view, the loss of the bone substance can either follow a horizontal or vertical/angular course.

Horizontal alveolysis generally represents the first etiopathogenic moment of periodontal disease, which can be described as follows: the bone, reducing its thickness in the cranio-caudal direction, causes the consequential damage of the alveolar ligament and the progressive uncovering of the neck and of the dental root. The latter sometimes keeps a partial gingival covering which can hide the process of bone destruction, which is easily evaluated through instrumental manoeuvres or radiologically. The horizontality of the process' progression is represented by the parallelism existing between the ridges of the residual proximal bone and an imaginary line traced along the cementoenamel junction (Fig. 6.6).

Concerning the radiological signs related to the aforementioned process, they are obviously extremely variable in relation to its evolutionary phase.

In the first phase, which can be considered relatively innocuous, alveolysis phenomena affect the apices of the **interdental crests** (Figs. 6.7 and 6.8).

The lysis of **interradicular crests** with exposure of **teeth furcations** is included in this stage, even if its finding is less frequent and is generally a sign of more severe situations (Fig. 6.9a, b)

The horizontal progression of the resorption process, further spreading to the spongiosa of the alveolar ridge, can evolve to degrees of extreme seriousness, where the bone depletion is associated to signs of severe instability in the dental elements.

As previously described, such situations give rise to the so-called **horizontal alveolar sockets**. In addition, radiological evaluation of such sockets is possible only when both the bone resorption bound and the gingival margin are visible (Fig. 6.10a, b).

Vertical or angular alveolysis has a course which is parallel or oblique with respect to the longitudinal axis of the tooth, and is fundamentally expressed by the formation of the so-called **infraosseous sockets** (Fig. 6.11a–c).

Infraosseous socket is a loss of osseous substance (which affects both the lamina dura and the adjacent spongiosa) limited to some of the dental elements. Therefore, it does not show the typical spread of horizontal alveolysis, with which, however, it is often variously associated.

From the pathological point of view, infraosseous sockets are categorised depending on the number of the bone walls which mark off their cavity. It is possible to identify four socket models with one, two or three walls or with circular walls (**niche socket**) (Fig. 6.12).

From the radiological perspective, such a distinction is not always possible, as the bidimensionality of the image allows it to provide documentary evidence only of the socket walls hit in profile by the radiant beam at the level of the mesial and/or distal side of the tooth. Conversely, lingual and vestibular walls of the socket are not analyzable (Fig. 6.13).

Therefore, the tridimensional CT axial acquisition represents the best methodology in order to achieve a complete evaluation of the infraosseous sockets.

To conclude this subject matter, it must be said that the distinction between vertical and horizontal alveolysis has importance above all for the didactic explanatory point of view, as the two entities are mutually and variably associated.

Therefore, the use of expressions such as '**mainly horizontal**' or '**mainly vertical**' **resorption** seems to be appropriate (Fig. 6.14).

Further progression of the periodontal structures' destruction causes what is considered to be the latest alteration of the process: the structural alteration of the apex and/or radicular axis of the dental element (**apicolysis/rhizolysis**).

This event recognises its genesis in the chronic suppurative flogosis, which, if prolonged for a long time, is able to cause the destruction of cementum and dentine, through the action of inflammation agents.

Such a process can sometimes be associated with a productive phenomenon with reparative meaning: the **reactive hypercementosis** (Fig. 6.15).

Suppurative origin of the aforementioned phenomenon is also shown by the possible detection of fistulous passageways which link the alveolitic inflammatory lesion to the mandibular canal (Figs. 6.16 and 6.17).

The final event of the periodontal apparatus' destruction process is represented by two phases: firstly, the complete disconnection and mobilisation of the dental element from the alveolar osteoligamentous supporting structures (Fig. 6.18a, b) and, secondly, the expulsion of the tooth till the complete **edentulia** of one or both maxillaries.

In such cases, the task of the radiological examination is not to quantitatively evaluate the thickness of the residual bone for implantological aims, but to provide documentary evidence of possible pathological situations which can interfere with the reconstructive planning (radicular residuals, inclusive elements, etc.) (Fig. 6.19).

Focal Periodontopathy or Periodontitis

Focal periodontitis is very similar to vertical alveolysis in those subjects whose periodontium is not totally affected. In fact this entity typically involves only one tooth.

It is characterised by a inflammatory and suppurative process of the periodontium, which recognises different pathogenetic mechanisms.

Microbial entrance in the periodontal apparatus can be caused by different factors:

- Contamination through alterations of the gingival closure, which can be secondary to incongruous manoeuvres, poor oral hygiene, endodontic treatment, prosthetic device, traumas, etc.
- Diffusion from a carious lesion (discendent diffusion) or a flogistic apical lesion (ascendant diffusion) (Fig. 6.20)

In these cases, radiographical semeiotic elements consist in the **periodontal space widening** (Fig. 6.21), at the initial phase of the process, and in the disappearance of the lamina dura and resorption of the perialveolar spongiosa when the disease has achieved serious stages (Figs. 6.22 and 6.23).

In more serious and inveterate cases, apico-rhizolysis signs and possible fistulisation phenomena with the mandibular canal can be detected. Sometimes, sclerosis of the adjacent spongiosa is recognised, too. This is the expression of reactive osteocondensation phenomena, to the osteitic process (Figs. 6.24, 6.25 and 6.26).

Periodontopathy Due to Loss of the Occlusal Load

This entity deserves to be considered separately, as it represents a pathological event related to the periodontal atrophy originating when a tooth loses its antagonist. This follows the absence of occlusal loading stimuli.

Therefore, the aforementioned condition constitutes a particular alteration of the periodontal apparatus in which infectious flogistic alterations do not play a key role, even if they can contribute to worsening the situation.

Radiographical signs mainly refer to the widening of the periodontal space with modest perialveolar demineralisation phenomena, in addition to the protrusion of the dental element towards the opposing arch (Fig. 6.27).

Image Gallery

Fig. 6.1 Very thin tartar spicular appositions (indicated by *arrows*) in the necks with minimal resorption phenomena of the interdental crests

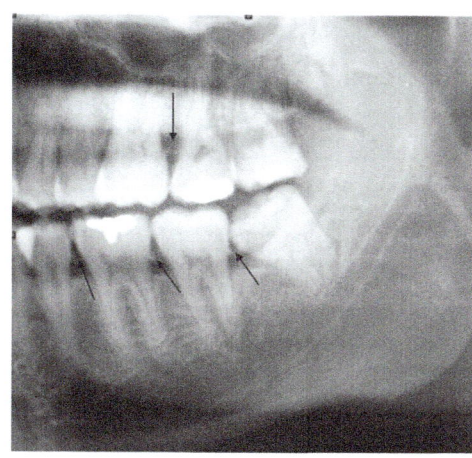

Fig. 6.2 Tartar spicular appositions (indicated by *arrows*) associated with serious resorption phenomena of the alveolar bone

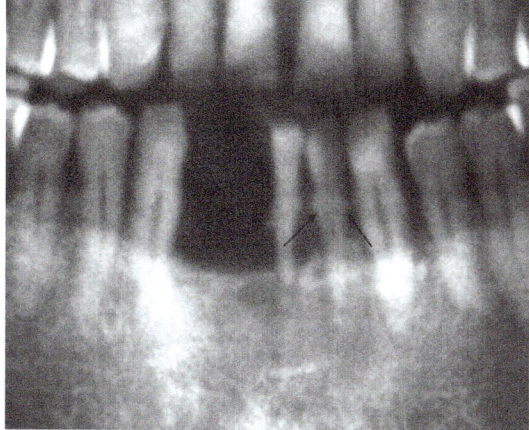

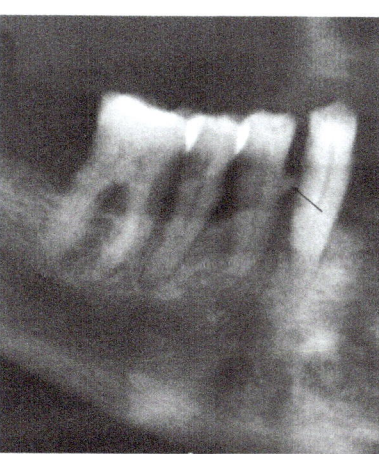

Fig. 6.3 Rough spicula (indicated by *arrow*) originating at radicular level

Fig. 6.4 Tartar apposition
with domed morphology
(indicated by *arrow*)

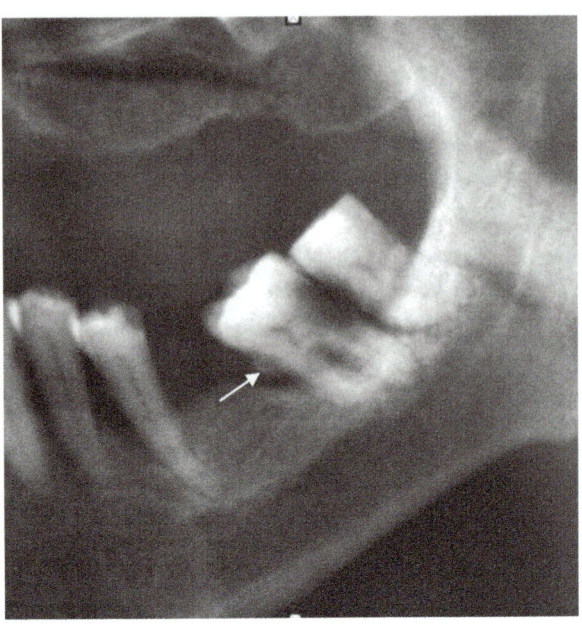

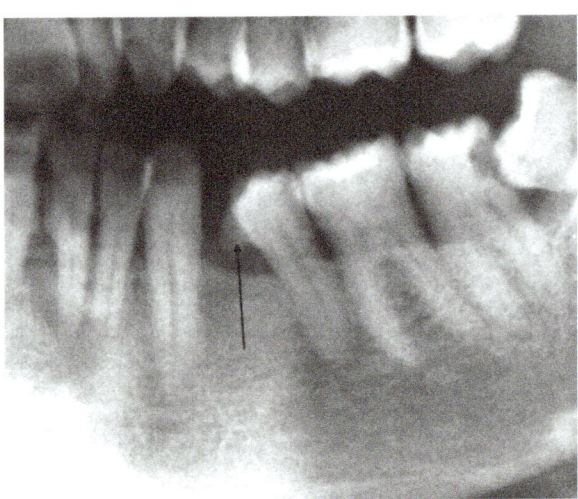

Fig. 6.5 Enormous tartar
spicula (*arrow*)

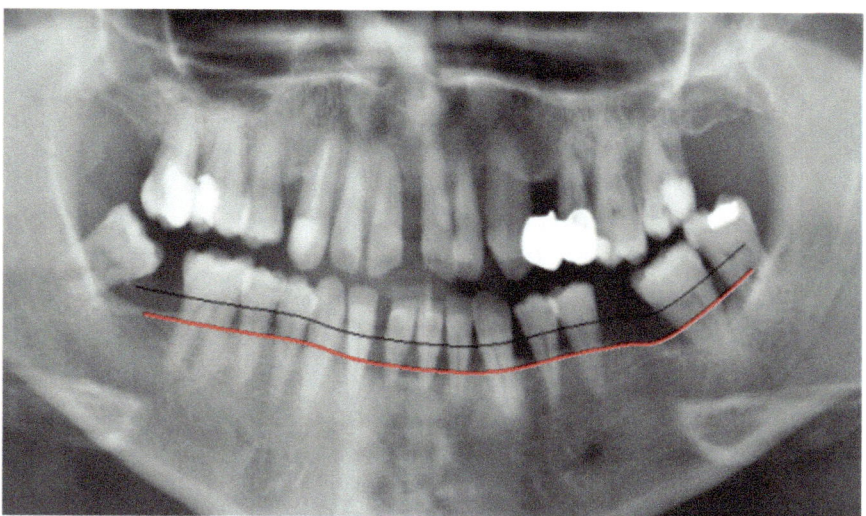

Fig. 6.6 Bone depletion with horizontal course. The *black line* indicates the cementoenamel junction. The *red line* indicates the front of the bone resorption

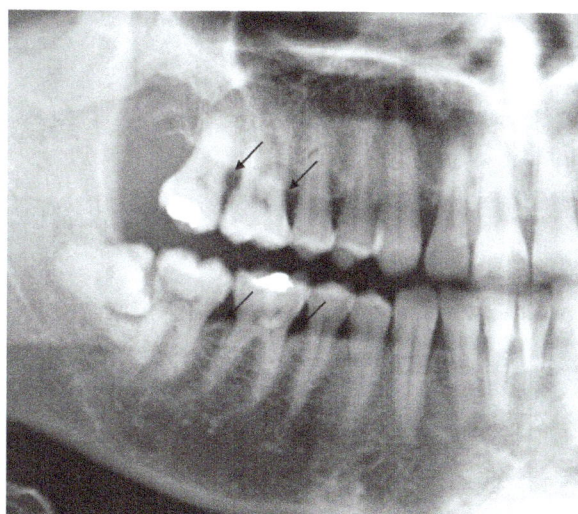

Fig. 6.7 Initial signs of bone resorption with rounded interdental crests (indicated by *arrows*)

Fig. 6.8 A more considerable bone resorption with respect to the previous figure. The front of the interdental crest's erosion appears concave (indicated by *short arrows*). Extended process of bone resorption and uncovered root of 1.3 (indicated by *long arrow*)

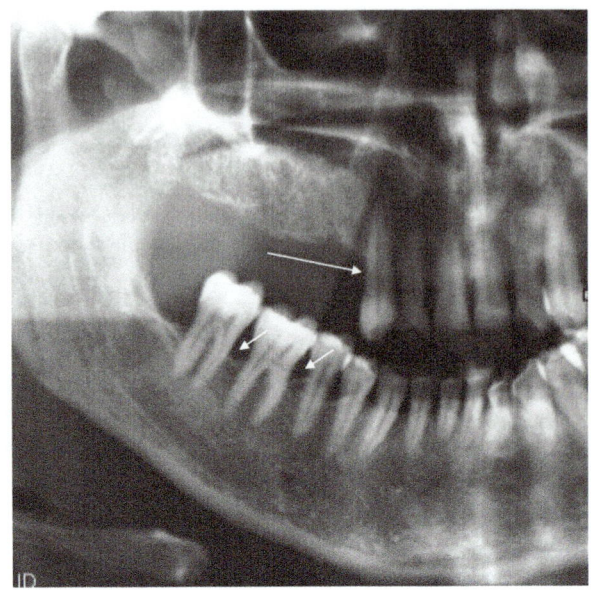

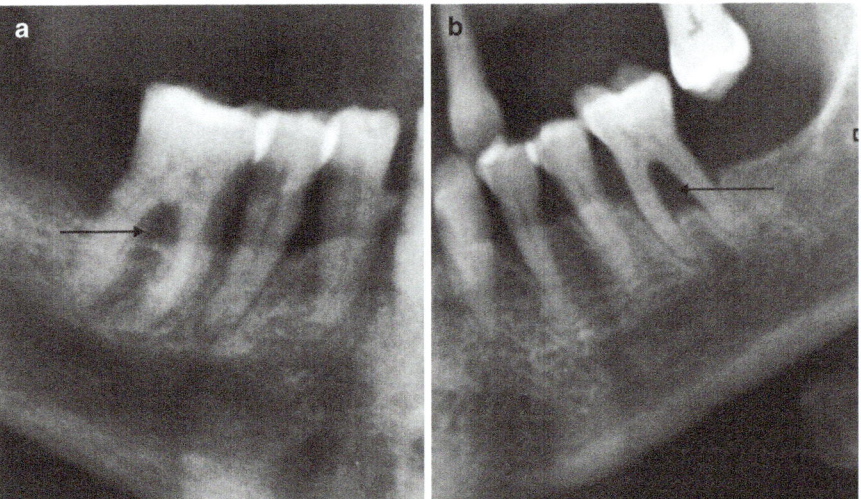

Fig. 6.9 Resorption of the interradicular crests (indicated by *arrows*). The alteration is almost visible in (**a**) and more marked in (**b**)

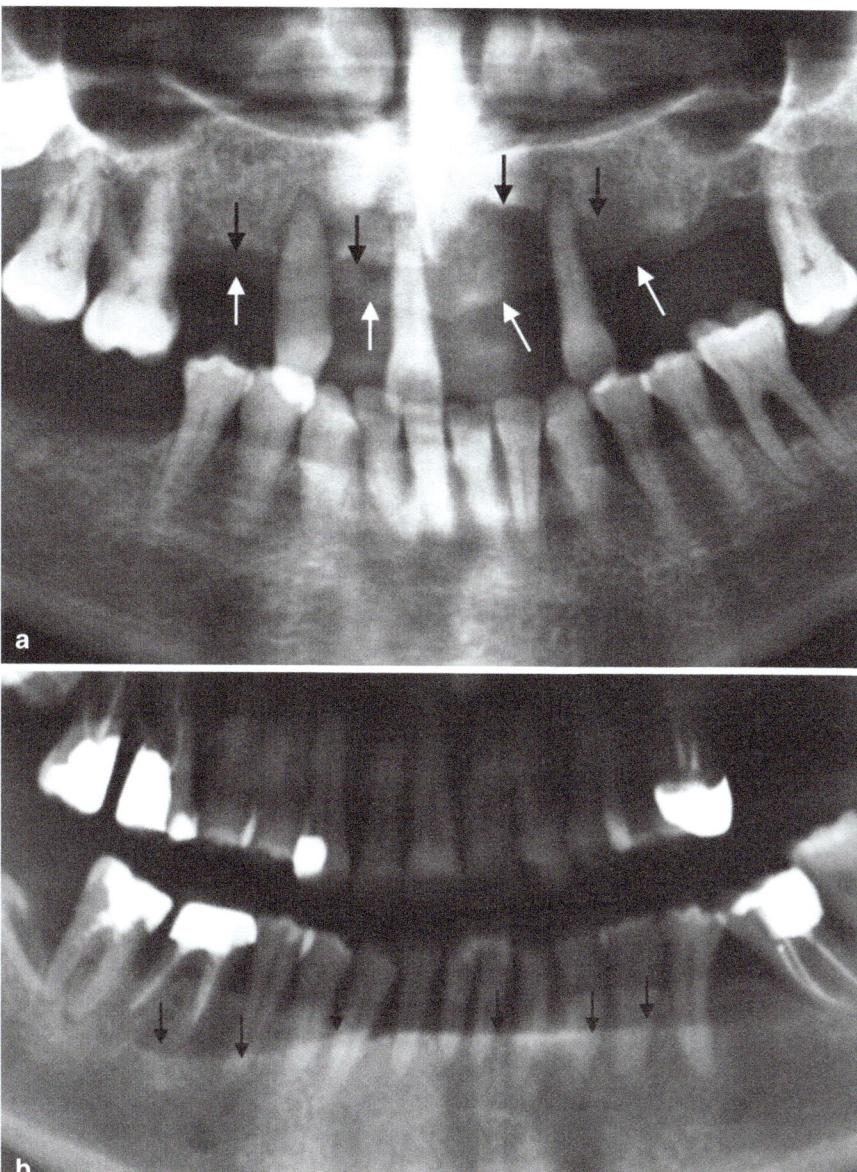

Fig. 6.10 (**a**) Finding of severe chronic periodontopathy. The *white arrows* indicate the gingival profile, while the *black arrows* indicate the front of bone resorption. The distance between the *black* and the *white arrows* indicate the depth of the horizontal socket which is particularly significant in the left superior hemiarch. (**b**) Horizontal socket of the inferior hemiarch. The *arrows* indicate the front of the bone's resorption

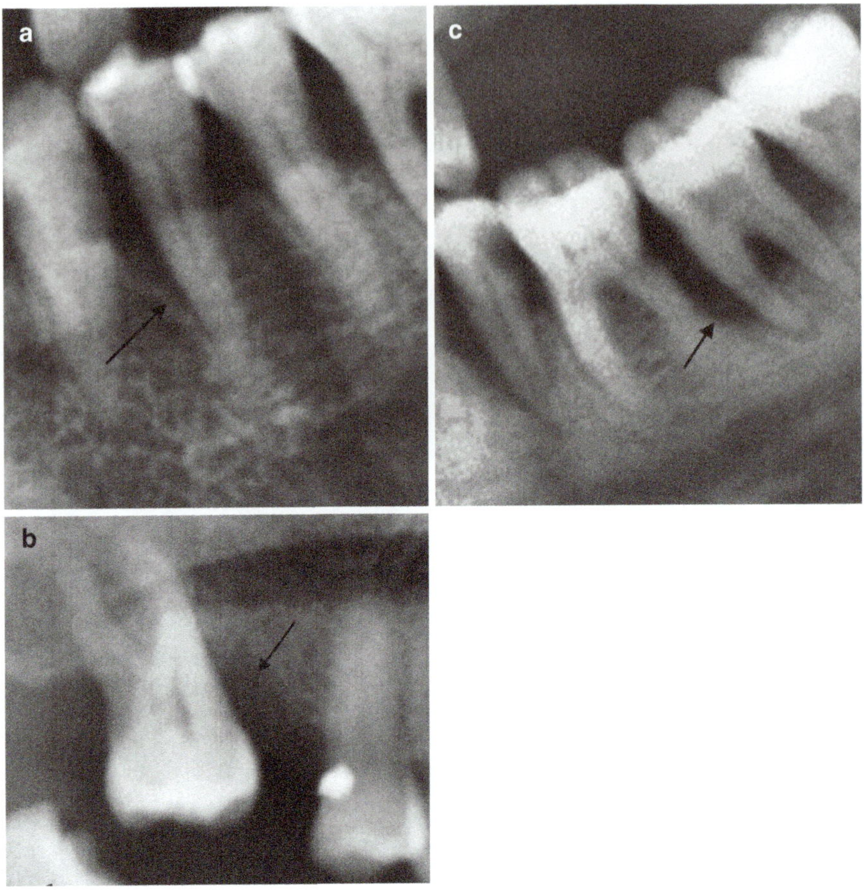

Fig. 6.11 (**a**–**c**) Vertical resorption. Infraosseous sockets of different extension and depth (indicated by *arrows*)

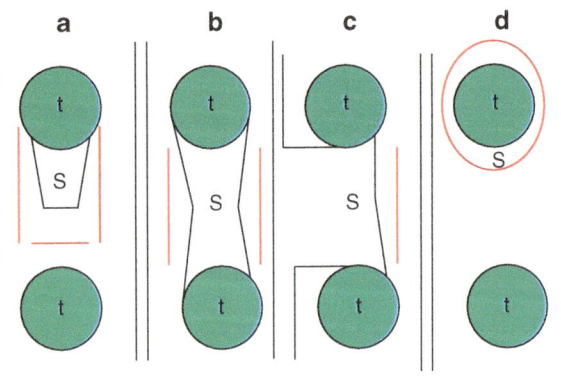

Fig. 6.12 Scheme illustrating the axial vision of the different types of infraosseous sockets (*S*). (**a**) Three wall socket. (**b**) Two wall socket. (**c**) One wall socket. (**d**) Round socket. The *red* lines indicate the residual bone walls of the socket. Letter *t* stands for 'teeth'

Fig. 6.13 The image shows infraosseous sockets: Socket of the element 4.6 seems to have a circular morphology as the whole alveolar bone structure is completely deleted. Socket of the element 4.4 has a morphology which is difficult to define. This is due to the presence of the residual bone which, because of the bidimensionality of the image, cannot be attributed with certainty to the lingual or vestibular wall of the alveolus

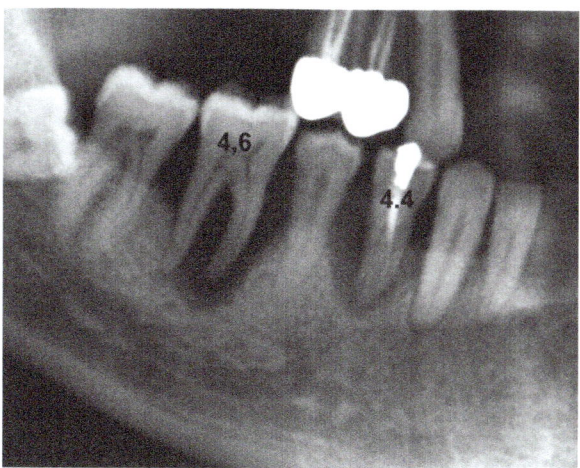

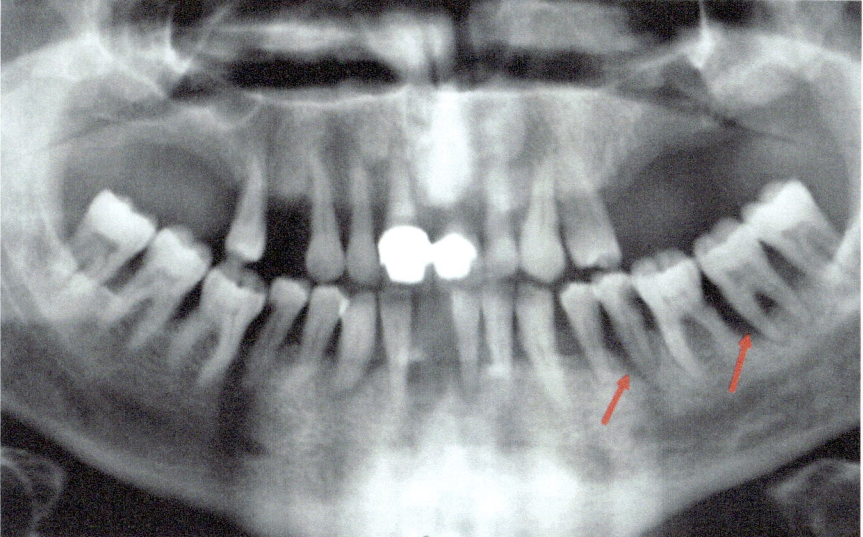

Fig. 6.14 Significant bone resorption mainly with horizontal course in both arcades, but with vertical course within the inferior left maxillary (indicated by *arrows*)

Fig. 6.15 Vertical alveolysis with reactive hyper-cementosis of the mesial root of 4.6 (see *arrow*)

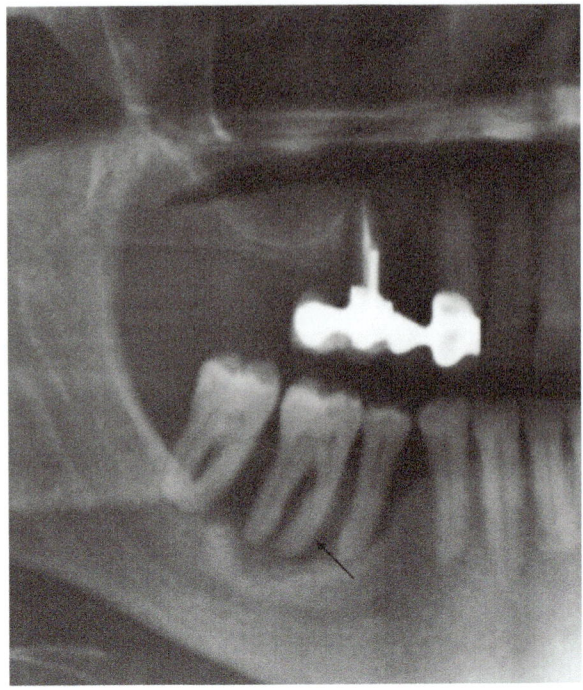

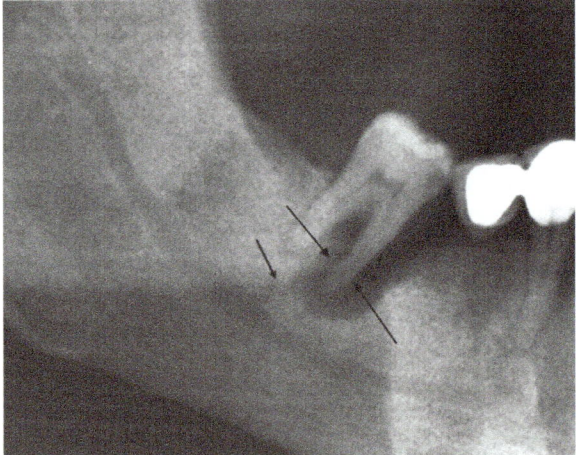

Fig. 6.16 Vertical alveolysis of 4.6 with initial signs of erosion of the mesial root's surface (indicated by *long arrows*). The *short arrows* indicates a subtle fistulous path towards the mandibular canal

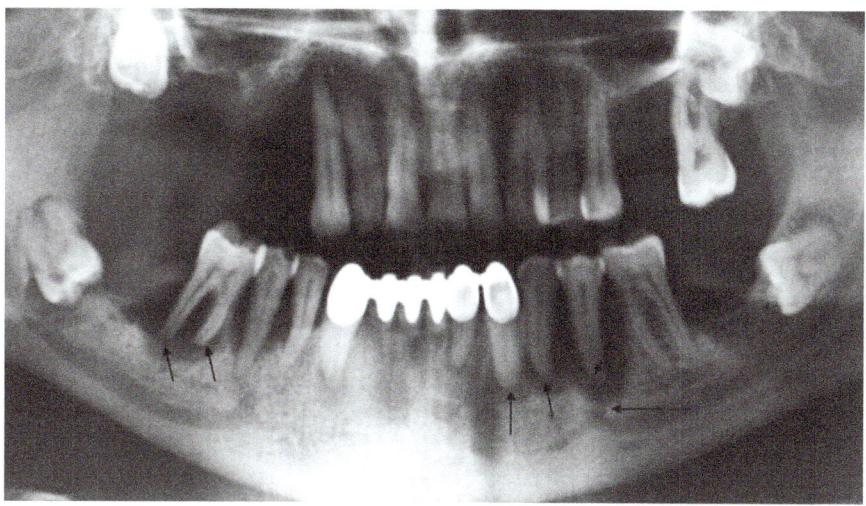

Fig. 6.17 Diffuse vertical alveolysis with apicolysis in numerous elements (indicated by the *short arrows*). Fistula with the mandibular canal (*long arrow*)

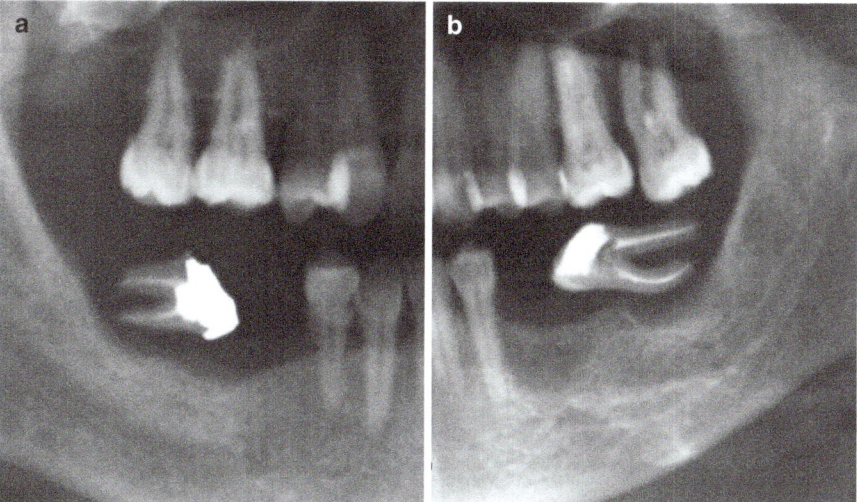

Fig. 6.18 (**a, b**) Disconnection and complete expulsive mobilisation of two elements

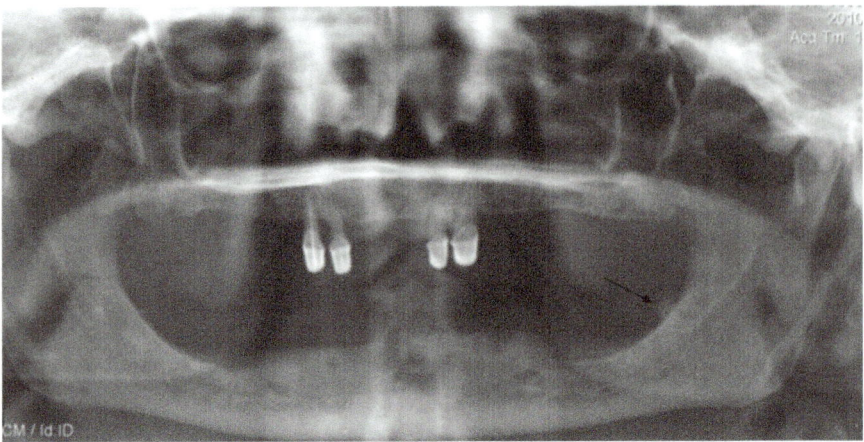

Fig. 6.19 Inferior arcade totally edentulous with radicular residual (indicated by *arrow*)

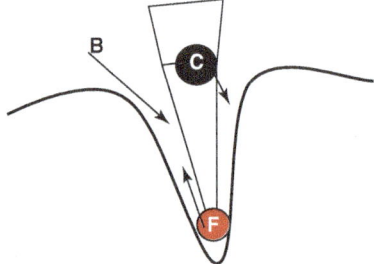

Fig. 6.20 Scheme illustrating the entrance ways of infection in the periodontal space. (*B*) From buccal cavity. (*C*) From carious lesion. (*F*) Periapical lesion

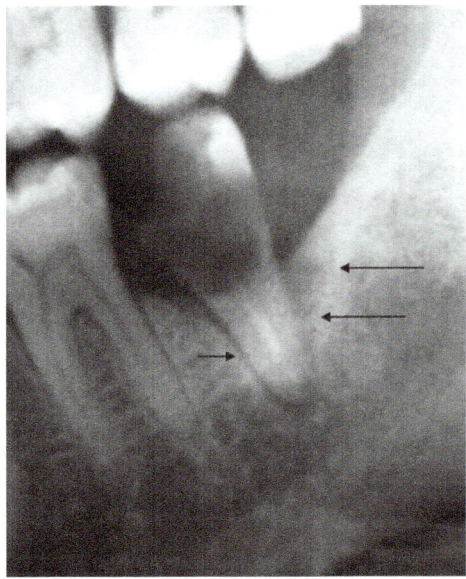

Fig. 6.21 Caries destroying the crown with widening of the periodontal space. In the mesial side, the lamina dura is still detectable (indicated by *short arrow*). In the distal side phenomena of bone resorption are present. They also extend towards the spongiosa (see *long arrows*)

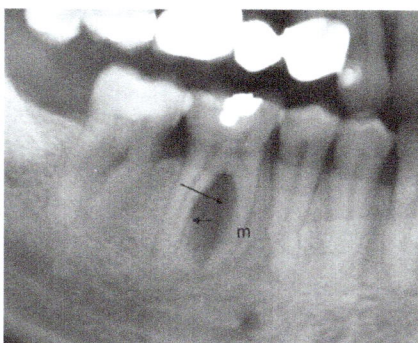

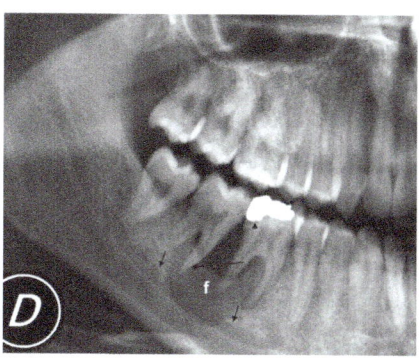

Fig. 6.22 The involvement of the periodontal space and the adjacent cancellous bone is present only in the interradicular side (the *short arrow* indicates the interruption of the lamina dura at the level of the distal root). The *long arrow* indicates the profile of the palatal root. Letter **m** indicates the mesial root

Fig. 6.23 Wide alveolitic lesion (*f*) with the loss of lamina dura, involving two adjacent elements. The *arrowhead* indicates recurrent, secondary caries of 4.6. The *long arrow* indicates the thinning of the mesial root's apex of 4.7. The effacement of the canal's edge bone (indicated by *short arrows*) indicates the involvement of the latter

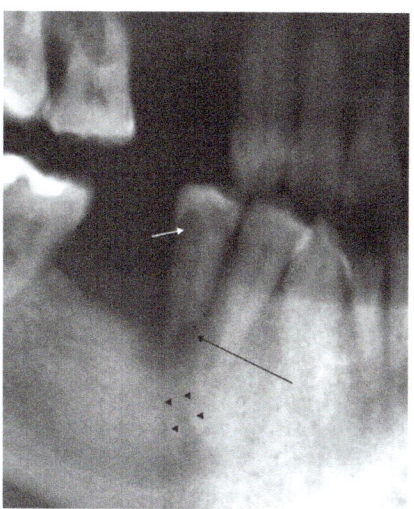

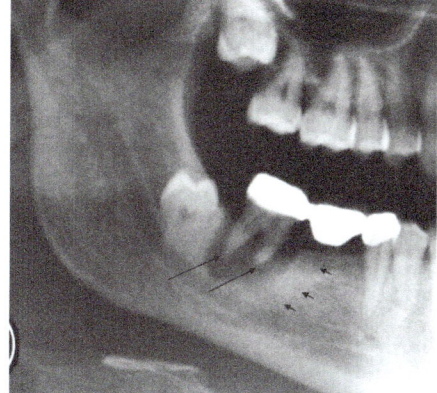

Fig. 6.25 Alveolysis in element being a pillar bridge. Apicolysis (indicated by *long arrows*) and sclerosis of the surrounding spongiosa (see *short arrows*)

Fig. 6.24 Caries of 4.5 (indicated by *white arrow*). Alveolysis with apicolysis (indicated by *long arrow*) and fistulisation towards the mandibular canal (indicated by *arrowheads*)

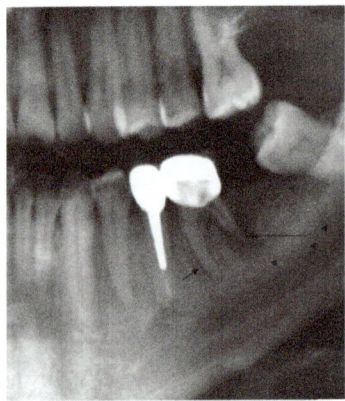

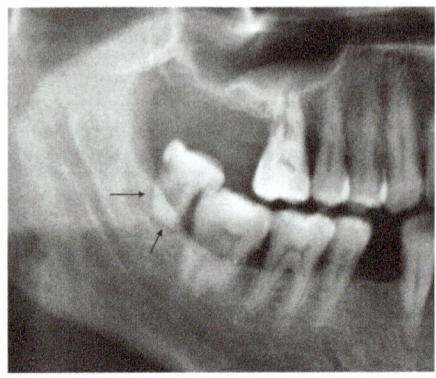

Fig. 6.26 Element with metal restoration of the crown. Phenomena of alveolysis and apicolysis of the distal root are present (indicated by *long arrow*). Sclerosis of the surrounding spongiosa (indicated by *arrowheads*). Slight widening of the periodontal space in the mesial root (indicated by *short arrow*)

Fig. 6.27 Loss occlusal load periodontopathy of 4.8. The element appears prominent and is characterised by the widening of the periodontal space (see *arrows*)

Suggested Reading

Awad EA, Al-Dharrab A (2011) Panoramic radiographic examination: a survey of 271 edentulous patients. Int J Prosthodont 24(1):55–57

Bergmans L, Van Cleynenbreugel J, Verken E et al (2002) Cervical external root resorption in vital teeth. J Clin Periodontol 29(6):580–585

Estrela C, Bueno MR, Leles CR, Azevedo B, Azevedo JR (2008) Accuracy of cone beam computed tomography and panoramic and periapical radiography for detection of apical periodontitis. J Endod 34(3):273–279

Hommez GM, De Meerleer GO, De Neve WJ, De Moor RJ (2012) Effect of radiation dose on the prevalence of apical periodontitis-a dosimetric analysis. Clin Oral Investig 16(6):1543–1547

Langland OE, Langlais R, Mc David W, Del Baso A (1989) Panoramic radiology, 2nd edn. Aufl, Lea & Febiger, Philadelphia

Leach HA (2001) Radiographic diagnosis of root resorption in relation to orthodontics. Br Dent J 190(1):16–22

Levander E et al (1998) Early radiographic diagnosis of apical root resorption during orthodontic treatment: a study of maxillary incisors. Eur J Orthod 20(1):57–63

Nab S et al (2000) External apical root resorption following orthodontic treatment. Angle Orthod 70(3):227–232

Nurbakhsh B, Friedman S, Kulkarni GV, Basrani B, Lam E (2011) Resolution of maxillary sinus mucositis after endodontic treatment of maxillary teeth with apical periodontitis: a cone-beam computed tomography pilot study. J Endod 37(11):1504–1511

Rinke S, Ohl S, Ziebolz D, Lange K, Eickholz P (2011) Prevalence of periimplant disease in partially edentulous patients: a practice-based cross-sectional study. Clin Oral Implants Res 22(8):826–833

Sameshima GT, Asgarifar KO (2001) Assessment of root resorption and root shape: periapical vs panoramic films. Angle Orthod 71(3):185–189

White SC, Pharoah MJ (2000) Oral radiology: principles and interpretation. Mosby, St Louis

Ziebolz D, Szabadi I, Rinke S, Hornecker E, Mausberg RF (2011) Initial periodontal screening and radiographic findings – a comparison of two methods to evaluate the periodontal situation. BMC Oral Health 11:3

Cystic Lesions and Maxillary Tumours

7

General Considerations on Cystic Lesions

Maxillary cystic lesions can be distinguished as having either odontogenic or non-odontogenic origin.

All odontogenic cystic lesions, except **radicular cysts**, present a dysontogenetic genesis which is variably linked to developmental errors of the dental germ and/or the organ of the enamel.

Radicular cysts are the only acquired odontogenic cysts which are mainly caused by a pre-existing inflammatory lesion (**apical granuloma**).

However, it must be said that flogistic phenomena do not exclusively pertain to radicular cysts, as the **dysontogenetic cysts** can also be complicated by possible inflammatory phenomena.

Non-odontogenic cysts always have a dysontogenetic origin, linked to the cystic degeneration of the epithelial residuals which, during the embrionary development, remained inclusive in specific areas of the maxillaries (**fissural cysts**).

Before treating the single pathological entities, it is appropriate to consider the so-called lacunar images of the mandible, which are included, often erroneously, in the category of cystic lesions.

Lacunar Images of the Mandible

This chapter includes lacunar images which are localised and clearly marked off by the surrounding bone and by a thin sclerotic rim, which can often be detected in the inferior maxillary.

Such a finding has been, for a long time, erroneously called 'Stafne's cysts'.

There is no doubt that the term 'cyst' is completely erroneous and used improperly as the genesis of such an image is not supported by fluid content, but rather by the intraosseous intrusion of a modest amount of tissue deriving from the parenchyma of the submandibular gland.

I. Pandolfo, S. Mazziotti, *Orthopantomography*,
DOI 10.1007/978-88-470-5289-5_7, © Springer-Verlag Italia 2013

This genesis explains the characteristic seat of the radiological image (mandibular angle region, beneath the mandibular canal) (Fig. 7.1a, b).

On the basis of what is aforementioned, it is clear that **Stafne's lacuna** is the most appropriate term to indicate such an image (moreover, without pathological meaning).

Radicular Cysts

Radicular cysts are the only odontogenic cysts with a primitive inflammatory origin.

Indeed, they are always supported by the presence of chronic flogistic phenomena localised in the periapical area or more rarely in the periradicular region.

In particular, it is believed that radicular cyst (apical or pararadicular) represents the cystic evolution of the epithelial remains (**Malassez' residuals**), which are included in the untreated apical (or pararadicular) granuloma.

For this reason, it must be remembered (as explained in the Chap. 5) that radiological differentiation between a big apical granuloma and a small cyst is based only on dimensional criteria, where the diameter of about 10–12 mm represents the limit between the two entities.

Radicular cysts are constituted by a cavity with slow growth, lined by an epithelial membrane and are characterised by a fluid content which tends to increase progressively. This is a consequence of the continuous osmotic uptake in the cavity.

The lesion is firstly asymptomatic, but in its growth, tumefactions in vestibular or lingual seat begin to appear.

Radicular or Periapical Cyst

In its periapical variety, the radicular cyst represents the most frequent cystic lesion.

It more frequently involves the anterior-lateral teeth of the superior maxillary and the posterior ones of the inferior maxillary.

It always shows itself on the apex of the pathological dental element, or in the seat of previous endodontic treatment (Fig. 7.2a–c).

Cystic localisations in the dental elements of the superior arch can be problematic because of such a particular seat of origin. A primary consideration which must be highlighted is the very close proximity of the cystic lesions to the maxillary sinuses.

This anatomical proximity can cause diagnostic errors (both positive and negative) which are linked to the difficulty of detecting the cyst, which can be confused with abnormal expansions of the sinus cavity (Fig. 7.3a, b and 7.4).

Another characteristic problem of the localised cysts in the superior arch is related to their possible endosinusal development.

Indeed, the growth of the cyst inside the maxillary sinus, above all if associated with calcification phenomena, can give rise to bizarre features of difficult interpretation (Fig. 7.5).

In the inferior maxillary the most significant problem related to the volumetric increase of the cystic lesion is represented by the existing relations between the latter and the mandibular canal.

Indeed, this proximity entails the risk of iatrogenic lesions in the inferior alveolar nerve during surgical manoeuvres aiming at treating the lesion.

In such a situation CT examination is obviously the method of choice as OPT is not sufficient to clarify in detail the existing relations between these structures.

Residual Radicular Cysts

This term indicates all the cyst cavities remaining after the tooth extraction.

In such cases the cavity can be totally asymptomatic or can continue in its growth, causing damages to the adjacent structures.

In the field of such lesion typology, it is possible to detect an extreme dimensional variability of the residual cavities which can vary from lesions of small dimension to substantially sized cysts (Figs. 7.6 and 7.7).

The diagnosis of a residual cyst, especially if it has huge dimensions, can be difficult and is exclusively based (apart from the anamnestic finding) on the radiological detection of the remains of the empty alveolus (Fig. 7.8).

Lateral Radicular Cysts

The **lateral radicular cyst** or **periradicular cyst** rarely occurs, and it stems from the cystic evolution of a **periradicular granuloma**, a pathological entity already discussed in Chap. 5.

It is easily diagnosticable when still characterised by modest volume (Fig. 7.9).

Conversely, in the presence of more extensive lesions affecting the adjacent dental elements, the diagnosis can be more difficult to make (Fig. 7.10).

Follicular or Dentigerous Cysts

The **follicular cyst**, also known as a **dentigerous cyst**, represents a classic type of odontogenic cyst on a non-inflammatory base.

Indeed, it is the expression of the cystic degeneration of the **enamel organ** and in particular of the **stellate reticulum** tissue (see Chap. 2) in an inclusive element.

The missing eruption, the seat of the dental element and variable alterations of its orientation therefore represent favourable circumstances for the development of a follicular cyst.

From the morphological point of view, the most characteristic element of such lesion is represented by the protrusion of the crown (more or less pronounced) inside the cystic cavity. Conversely, the radicular axis generally turns out to be on its exterior.

The third molars, followed by the canines (most likely for their major tendency to inclusion), are the most affected teeth.

Radiologically the follicular cyst presents an extreme variability, and its innumerable variations can be noticed both in terms of localisation and dimension.

With respect to this, it must be said that the lesions characterised by modest size (which represent the majority of the radiological findings) are generally asymptomatic and are detected only occasionally (Figs. 7.11a–c and 7.12a, b).

Conversely, the more extensive lesions can have a clinical evidence for three reasons: the presence of tumefaction and deformity of the skeletal host segment, its relations to the surrounding critical structures (paranasal sinuses and mandibular canal) and, finally, the damages occurring in the adjacent normal dental elements (Fig. 7.13a, b).

The Eruption Cyst

It is a variant of the follicular cyst characterised by the presence of **pericoronal cystic degeneration** in an element which is totally or partially inclusive but whose orientation (normal or only slightly altered) presupposes its eruption.

In these cases, if the eruptive push prevails on the resistance exerted by the cystic cavity, eruption occurs.

The eruption cyst clinically appears as a bluish swelling covered by the gingival mucosa, whose laceration reveals the tooth in eruptive phase (Fig. 7.14a, b).

Primordial Cyst and Odontogenic Keratocyst

For their similarity these two entities are considered to be variants of the same pathological phenomenon.

Moreover, both lesions have odontogenic origin.

Primordial cyst is the expression of the cystic degeneration of a dental germ, before the latter becomes mineralised.

The dental germ which is affected corresponds a normal or a supernumerary element.

Obviously, in the first case, the absence of a dental element (generally one of the molars) will correspond to the cystic lesion.

Conversely, in the second eventuality the lesion will coexist with all the elements of the permanent dentition.

Odontogenic keratocyst is related to the cystic degeneration of a portion of the dental lamina, in a greater or lesser extent.

Therefore, from the embryologic point of view, it is an older lesion than the primordial cyst. As a matter of fact, some authors categorise it in the field of hamartomas.

The distinctive structural feature of this lesion involves the presence of a keratinised epithelial lining.

Similarly to the primordial cyst, it can develop when the elements of the permanent dentition are normally represented or when absence of a permanent dental element occurs.

Both lesions typically occur in the mandibular angular region and are obviously mutually not distinguishable.

The radiological aspect, which is totally nonspecific, is constituted by a lytic lesion which can be monocameral or with thin sepiments in its interior, delimited by a thin and regular sclerotic rim (Fig. 7.15a, b).

During their growth, lesions can displace the adjacent dental elements, sometimes enveloping them.

In this case, the differential diagnosis of an unusual follicular cyst can be difficult and even impossible to make.

The angular region of the mandible is also the typical seat where numerous varieties of odontogenic tumours originate. Therefore, it is evident that the cystic lesions with conspicuous dimensions and which cause dislocation or damage to the adjacent dental elements are difficult or impossible to distinguish from possible neoplasms such as the **monolocular ameloblastoma**.

Odontogenic Tumours

Odontogenic tumours are generally constituted by benign or mildly aggressive entities, even if they often tend towards local relapse.

These neoformations are presented together with the cystic lesions, as the odontogenic tumours, even if rare, show considerable overlaps with the more common cystic formations, both on clinical and radiological levels. However, there are some exceptions, such as odontomas.

Consequently it must be said that most of the time, the clinical/radiological differential diagnosis between an odontogenic tumour and an odontogenic cyst is almost impossible.

In fact, the final pathological diagnosis is often a revelation in those patients who arrive at the operating table with a presumptive diagnosis of a cystic lesion.

Nosographic classification of the odontogenic tumours is usually determined on the basis of the tissue of origin (epithelium, mesenchyma or both) and on the degree of differentiation.

Table 7.1, even if in a fairly simplistic and general way, summarises this conception.

Odontoma

Odontomas represent the most frequent odontogenic tumours.

The term 'odontoma' includes well-differentiated neoplasms and those having mixed derivation (both epithelial and mesenchymal) which consequently originate from all the tissue components of the tooth (dentine, enamel, cementum).

Table 7.1 Table summarizing the classification of odontogenic tumours

	Epithelial	Mixed	Mesodermal
Differentiated	Adenomatoid odontogenic tumor	Odontoma	Calcifying cystic odontoma
	Squamous odontogenic tumor		
Mixed	Calcifying odontogenic cyst		
	Calcifying epithelial odontogenic tumor (Pindborg)		
Undifferentiated	Ameloblastoma	Ameloblastic fibroma	Myxoma

In this field it is possible to distinguish between **simple odontomas**, which are constituted by a single tissue component, and those having a complex structure.

Lesions which are constituted only by the dentine are indicated with the term of **dentinomas**. These are radiologically represented by small granulous formations, which are intensely radiopaque, often in relation to the occlusal surface of a tooth (Fig. 7.16a, b).

Lesions originating from the enamel constitute small aggregates; they are also characterised by high opacity and are adjacent to the surface of the dental element (**pearls of the enamel**).

Lesions originating from the cementum (**cementomas**), whose neoplastic nature is still doubtful, have already been discussed in Chap. 5.

Odontomas constituted by all the tissue components generate two main radiological features.

The so-called **complex odontoma** appears as a nodular image, intensely radiopaque, with amorphic structure in which the three components are variably mixed and not discernible (Fig. 7.17).

Conversely, **compound odontoma** appears as an agglomerate of small nodular elements, with granulous aspect, referable to small rudimental dental germs.

The aforementioned granulous images turn out to be closely bound up and are delimited by a thin radiolucent rim (Fig. 7.18a, b).

Some authors have compared this characteristic image to a bag filled with marbles (**marble bag**).

Both dentinomas and complex or compound odontomas often impede the normal dental eruption. Therefore, they can often be associated to phenomena of dental retention.

Adenomatoid Odontogenic Tumour (Ameloblastic Odontogenic Tumour)

The **adenomatoid odontogenic tumour** (**AOT**) is an extremely rare entity which is included in the well-differentiated lesions, but, in contrast to the odontomas, has an exclusively epithelial origin.

This is a lesion typically occurring in young subjects (second decade) characterised by a radiolucent and simil-cystic area, with sharp outlines. In 75 % of cases it contains the crown of an inclusive element.

It is clear that in such cases the lesion is substantially indistinguishable from a common follicular cyst, except when calcifications, especially evident in its peripheral portion, occur (Fig. 7.19).

If the inclusive element is not present, the lesion is indistinguishable from all the expansive formations in the maxillaries which present themselves as an osteolytic lesion with sharp outlines.

Squamous Odontogenic Tumour

The **squamous odontogenic tumour** (**SOT**) also represents a rare neoformation in the field of well-differentiated lesions with epithelial origin. It is absolutely benign and typically occurs in young adults.

It is frequently localised in the anterior region of the superior maxillary and the posterior area of the mandible.

It is a tumour which creates osteolytic and simil-cystic images, totally nonspecific, often adjacent to the radicular axis of an element. They can appear variably altered, due to the presence of an expansive lesion, but always in a dental element which is sane and vital in the other aspects (Fig. 7.20).

This last observation represents a criterion for which the diagnosis of the radicular cyst (generally associated to an altered tooth) would at least be questioned.

Calcifying Epithelial Odontogenic Tumour

The **calcifying epithelial odontogenic tumour** (**CEOT**), also known as **Pindborg tumour**, is a moderately differentiated neoplasm with epithelial origin, in which an amorphic substance similar to the amyloid is present. It does not occur in a specific age, but it seems to be more frequent in young adults.

The neoplasia usually occurs in the posterior region of the mandible and is clinically and macroscopically very similar to the most common ameloblastoma from which, in its pure osteolytic forms, is not radiographically distinguishable.

The presence of extended calcification within the lesion can be a clue for orientating the diagnosis (Fig. 7.21).

Calcifying Odontogenic Cyst

The term **calcifying odontogenic cyst** (**COC**) or **Gorlin cyst** indicates an heterogeneous set of lesions characterised by histological finding of keratinised cells (**ghost cells**).

This kind of lesion frequently onsets, but not exclusively, in the second decade of life.

At the beginning, it is osteolytic and characterised by central development. Conversely in one third of the cases, it can present as an esophytic lesion with respect to the host bone.

In its interior it often shows an inclusive element; therefore, in its pure osteolytic phase, it is very similar to a common dentigerous cyst.

In the calcifying phases, more or less extended, the diagnosis of the Gorlin cyst can be taken into account.

Ameloblastoma

The **ameloblastoma** or **adamantinoma** is an epithelial lesion in which the cell lineage is similar to the one present in the **organ of the enamel**, even if with immature aspects.

The lesion affects youths (only one third of such lesions is diagnosed after 40 years old). The majority of localisations (about 80 %) occurs in the mandible.

The radiological expressions of the lesion are nonspecific, and, in the majority of cases, they appear as an osteolytic image with geographical outlines. The lesion swells the bone segment, to a greater or lesser extent, with interruption of the corticals in the most conspicuous lesions.

Sometimes (in about 20 % of cases), the presence of an intralesional inclusive element can be documented.

It is obvious as, on the basis of these considerations, the radiological differential diagnosis of dentigerous cyst, along with other odontogenic tumours, turns out to be difficult, sometimes impossible to make.

The sepimented and multicameral (**multilocular ameloblastoma**) aspect of the osteolysis (Figs. 7.22, 7.23 and 7.24) is more specific and therefore indicative of the presence of an ameloblastoma.

Among the odontogenic tumours, ameloblastoma is one of the most frequent lesions. It is characterised by a slow growth, but with a certain tendency towards local invasiveness which turns out to be the cause of possible relapses.

With respect to the aforementioned entities related to the odontogenic tumours, it follows that the radiologist must be aware of the presence of focal osteolytic lesions while making an OPT report.

It is clear that, probabilistically, in the presence of a lytic lesion on the apex of an altered tooth or a lesion containing the crown of a dental element, the most obvious and realistic diagnosis will be respectively related to a **radicular cyst** and a **follicular cyst**.

Such a consideration, even if dictated by common sense, does not justify an uncritical diagnosis of 'cyst' because neoplastic entities containing and/or relating to the dental elements are numerous.

Using the formula 'compatible with cystic lesion' seems to be prudential.

Histological examination and other techniques (CT and MR) provide better information concerning the characteristics of the lesion and are necessary in order to make a correct final diagnosis.

The detection of lytic lesions, with the presence of more or less extended calcifications, also represents a nonspecific finding, even if allowing the restriction of hypothesis to a more reduced number of lesions.

Non-odontogenic Cysts

Fissural Cysts

Non-odontogenic cysts are also known as fissural cysts.

This denomination refers to the origin of the lesions. Indeed, they arise from cystic degeneration of epithelial residuals which, during embryonic development, remained inclusive between the constituents of the maxillary skeleton.

On the basis of what is aforementioned, fissural cysts can be distinguished between **median cysts** (precisely developing in the midline of skeletal structures which are mutually symmetrical) and **paramedian cysts**.

Incisive canal cysts or **nasopalatine cyst**, the more rare **median fissural cyst** and also the less frequent **mandibular median cyst** are included in the first variety (Figs. 7.25, 7.26a, b and 7.27).

The **globulomaxillary cyst** is the most known of the **fissural paramedian cysts**.

The incisive canal cyst is the most frequent among fissural cysts. It onsets along the nasopalatine canal, developing between the two median superior incisors.

Because the cyst can produce a variable increasing of the distance between the teeth, it should be considered one of possible cause of **diastema**.

The incisive canal cyst can be totally asymptomatic, or appear as a small soft-elastic tumefaction at the level of the **incisive papilla**.

The **median fissural cyst** can be localised either more cranially or more posteriorly to the latter as it originates from the epithelial residuals which remained inclusive between the articular surfaces of the palatine processes of the maxillary.

Therefore, it does not present significant anatomical relationship with the incisor elements.

The **globulomaxillary cyst** represents a paramedian fissure cyst coming from the epithelial residuals which remained inclusive between the maxillary and its nasal process.

Therefore, it is typically localised between the lateral incisor and the canine which consequently result variably displaced (Fig. 7.28a, b).

Globulomaxillary cyst can be included in the differential diagnosis with a possible radicular cyst, as the aforementioned lesions can frequently appear in such a seat.

A globulomaxillary cyst can be distinguished from a radicular cyst because it generally affects sane and vital elements, while radicular cysts are always associated to variably pathological dental elements.

Less significant is the dislocation model of the dental elements, which, if typical of the globulomaxillary cyst, can occasionally occur in the presence of radicular cysts.

Non-odontogenic Tumours of the Maxillaries

Neoplastic localisations in the maxillaries can be distinguished between primitive tumour lesions with osteomedullary origin (**osteoma, osteosarcoma, chondrosarcoma, myeloma**, etc.) and **secondary neoplasms of the maxillaries** such as the hematogenous metastasis or the tumours which affect the maxillaries for their adjacency, for example, the lesions in the oral cavity and of the salivary glands.

Finally, another category is represented by rare neoplasms which originate from the alveolar inferior nerve.

In this chapter not all the primitive tumours of the maxillaries and the metastasis will be discussed, because their radiological features are similar to those of the localisations of such diseases in other skeletal districts.

This is also due to the fact that OPT is not a procedure generally employed for the oncologic evaluation of patients with such tumours.

Conversely, secondary lesions, tumour propagation from the oral cavity to the maxillary and the rare neoplasias originating from the alveolar nerve will be mentioned.

Secondary Tumours of the Maxillaries

These are alterations of the skeletal components of the maxillaries. They are totally nonspecific but can easily be detected by the radiologist as long as he is aware of the patient's clinical situation.

They are generally epithelial neoplasias originating from the mucosa of the different sub-seats of the oral cavity, such as the **gingival mucosa**, the **retromolar trigone** and **the buccal floor** (Figs. 7.29 and 7.30).

Neoplasms originating from the **major** or (more often) **minor salivary glands**, such as the **adenoid cystic carcinoma**, can also affect the maxillaries. They are characterised by a diffusion along the inferior alveolar nerve (**perineural diffusion**) which is radiographically represented by the widening of the mandibular canal (Fig. 7.31a, b).

In osteolytic lesions, which occur more frequently, the normal architecture of the cortex and cancellous bone is deeply altered.

Osteosclerotic alterations can also exist along with the involvement and tumefaction of the soft tissues which cause avulsion and instability of the dental elements.

Anamnestic and especially inspective evaluation is needed by the radiologist to detect these alterations, as similar alterations can also occur in non-neoplastic condition, such as **osteomyelitis** and **necrosis due to phosphonates**.

Finally, lesions originating from the inferior alveolar nerve radiographically appear as alterations of the mandibular canal, because they stem from the vascular-nervous content of the canal itself.

Therefore, the neoplasias of this district will generally be of neurogenic origin (**schwannomas**) and of vascular origin (**angiomas**, **arteriovenous fistulas**, etc.) (Figs. 7.32 and 7.33).

Image Gallery

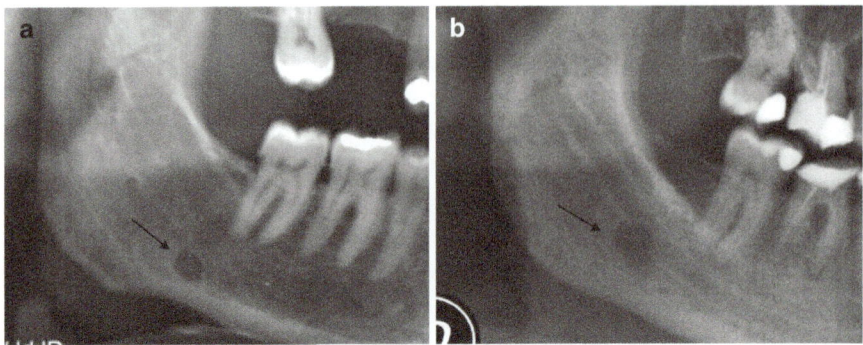

Fig. 7.1 (**a**, **b**) Two cases of Stafne's lacuna (indicated by *arrows*)

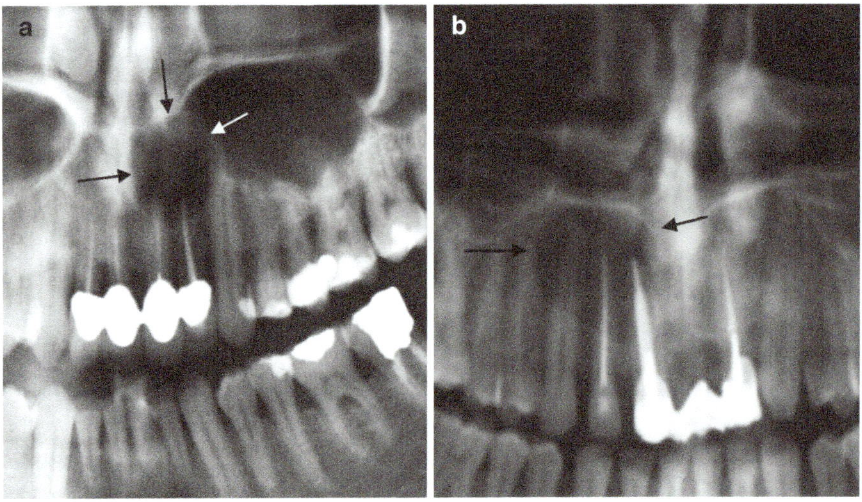

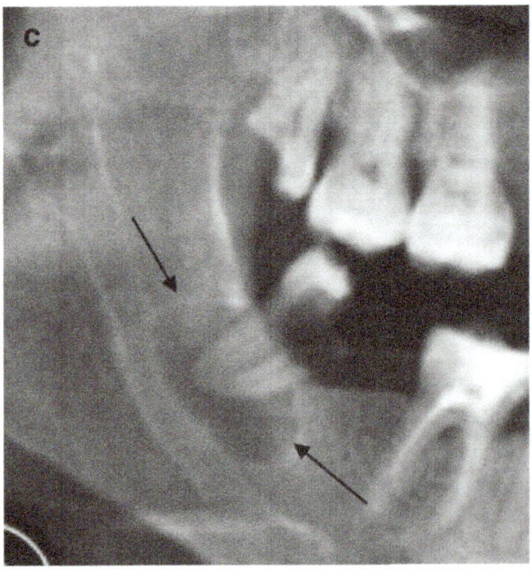

Fig. 7.2 (**a**, **b**) Radicular cysts (indicated by *arrows*) centred in the apical region of devitalised elements. (**c**) Radicular cyst (indicated by *arrows*) centred in the apex of an element with penetrating caries

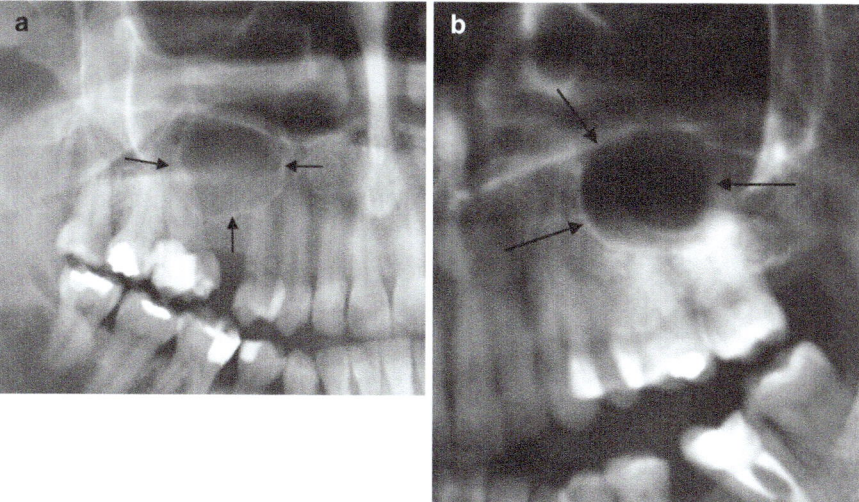

Fig. 7.3 (**a, b**) Two cases of abnormal expansion of the maxillary sinus (indicated by *arrows*) which can be confused with the presence of radicular cysts

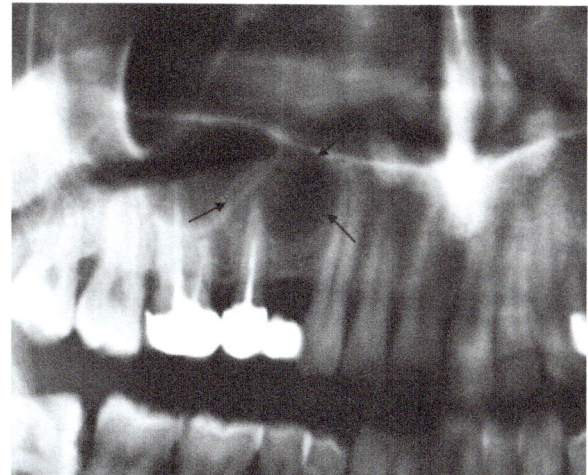

Fig. 7.4 Radicular cysts (indicated by *arrows*) centred in the apex of 1.5, which can be confused with the abnormal expansion of the maxillary sinus

Fig. 7.5 Calcified radicular
cyst with intrasinusal
development (indicated by
arrows)

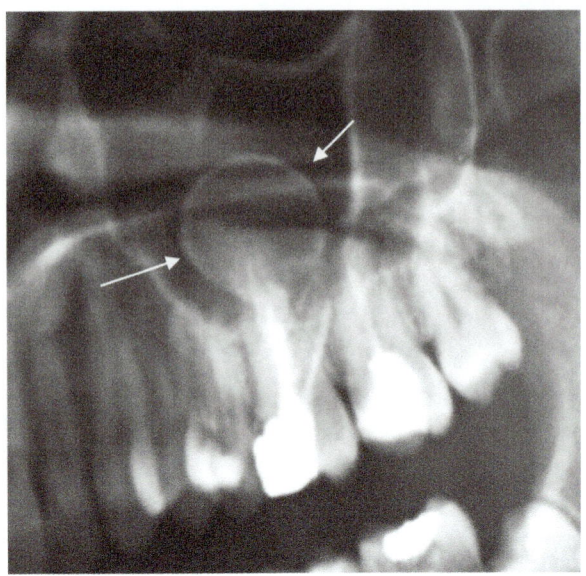

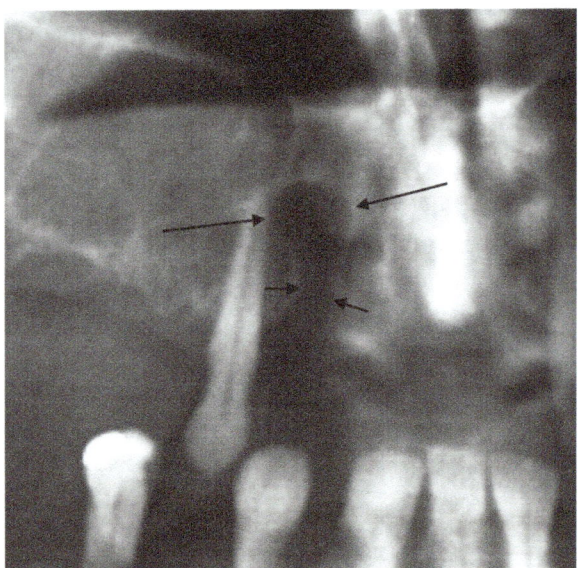

Fig. 7.6 Residual radicular
cyst (indicated by *long
arrows*). The *short arrows*
indicate the empty dental
alveolus

Fig. 7.7 Conspicuous residual cyst (indicated by *arrows*) developing in the maxillary sinus

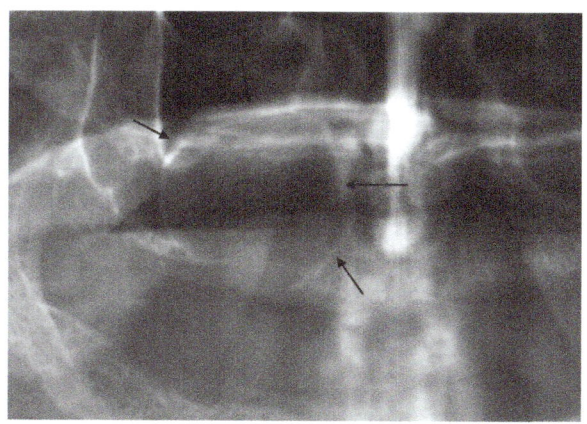

Fig. 7.8 Extended cystic lesion (indicated by *arrows*) which causes apicolysis of two elements. The residual nature of the lesion is shown by the detection of a subtle path (indicated by *short arrow*) which corresponds to the empty alveolus

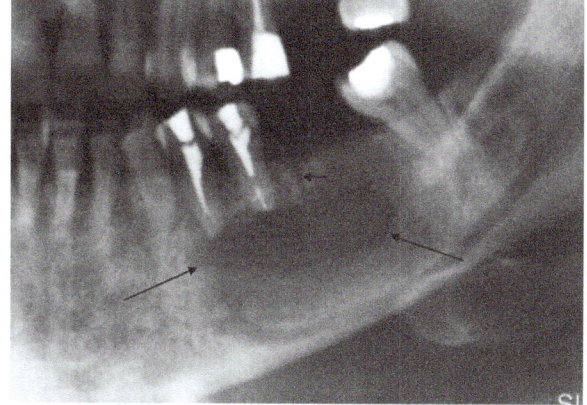

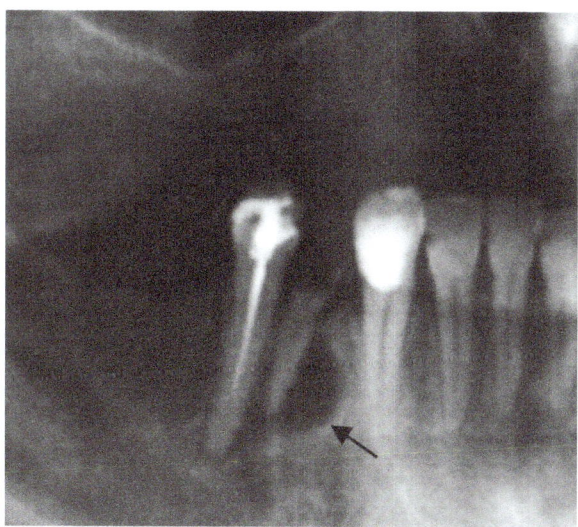

Fig. 7.9 Small radicular lateral cyst (indicated by *arrow*)

Fig. 7.10 Radicular lateral cyst of 2.1 (indicated by *arrows*) which, in its development overlaps 2.2, simulating its origin in this last element, which moreover, does not have any pathology

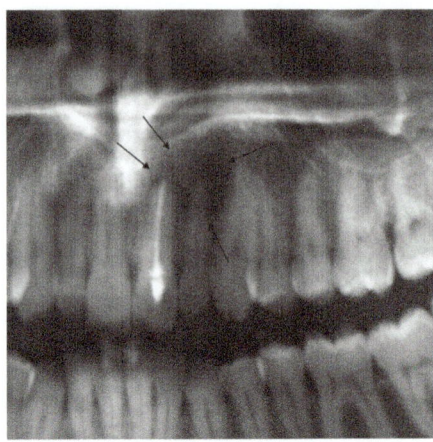

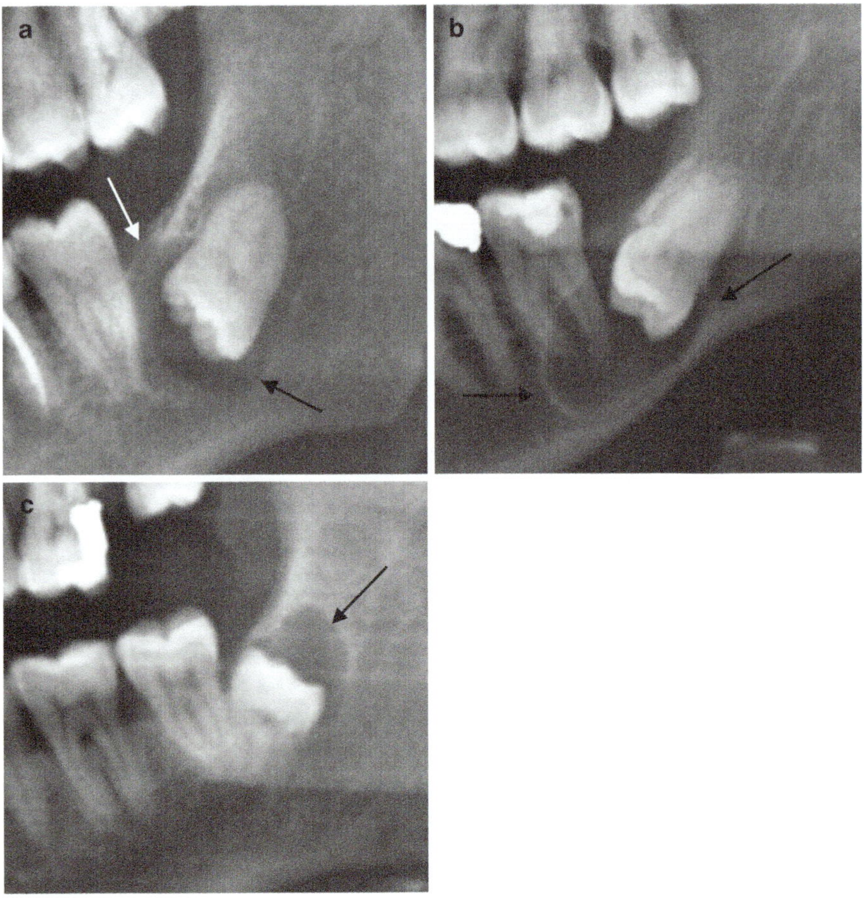

Fig. 7.11 (**a–c**) Three examples of small follicular cysts (indicated by *arrows*) of occasional finding

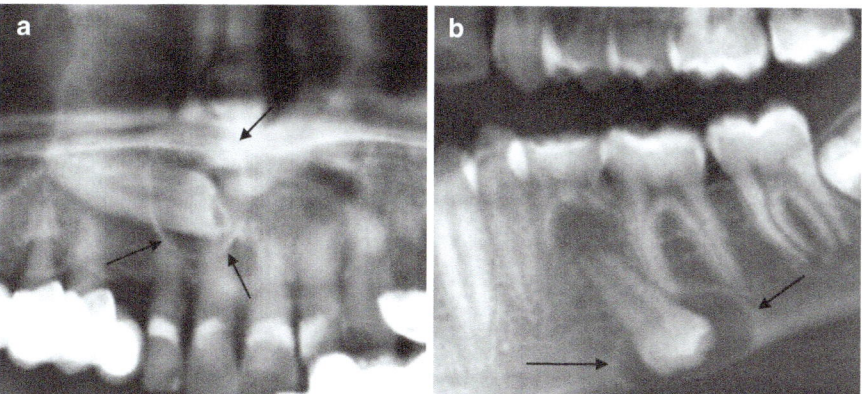

Fig. 7.12 (a) 1.3 is inclusive in mesiodistal angulation with a small follicular cyst (indicated by *arrows*). (b) Inclusive tooth in inverted orientation with a follicular cyst (indicated by *arrows*) which causes the thinning of the mandibular cortical is 3.5. Persistence of 7.5

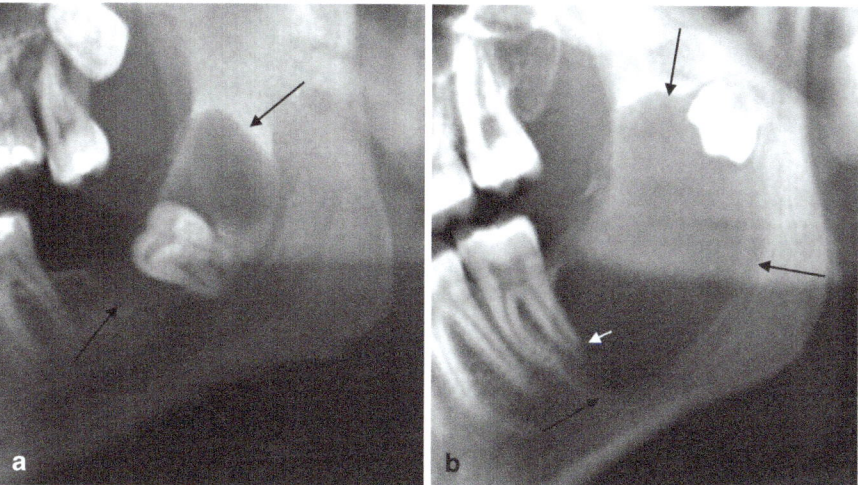

Fig. 7.13 (a, b) Conspicuous follicular cysts (indicated by *long arrows*). Both lesions present an extended surface of contact with the mandibular canal. Cyst in (b) also causes apicolysis of 3.7 (indicated by the *short arrow*)

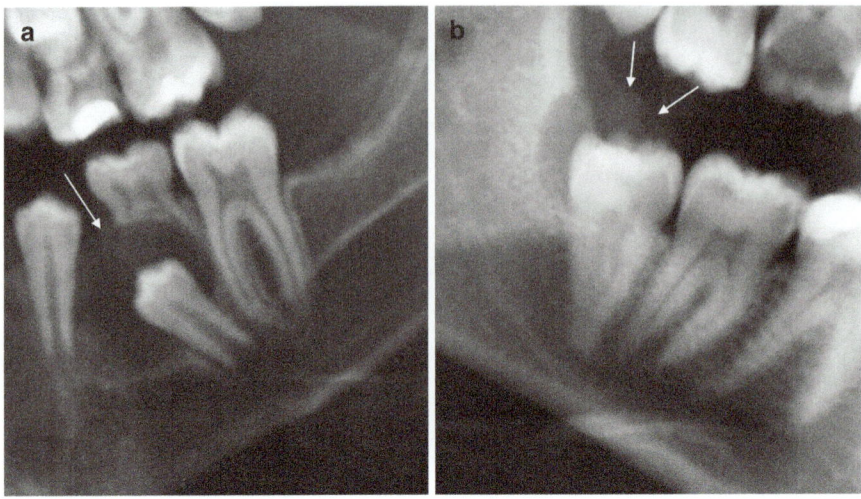

Fig. 7.14 (**a, b**) Two examples of eruption cysts. The *arrows* indicate the surface of the lesions appearing in the gum

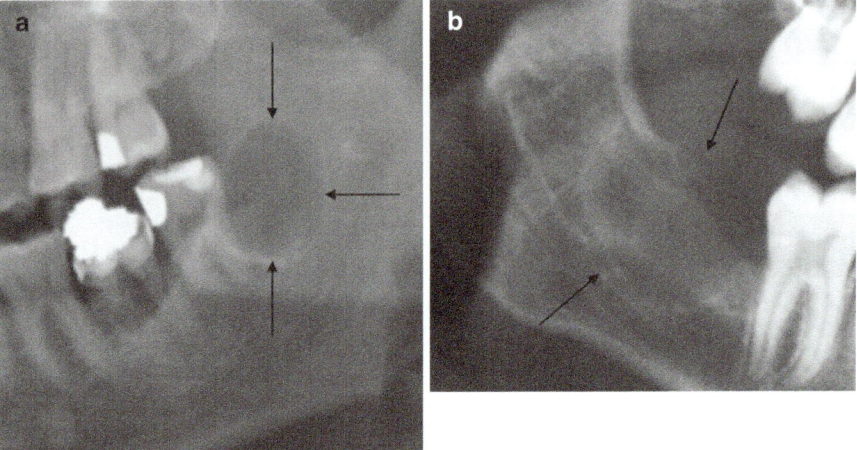

Fig. 7.15 (**a, b**) Two cases of primordial cysts (indicated by *arrows*) in mandibular angular region. In **a** the cyst derives from a supernumerary element. In (b) the cysts replaces two elements

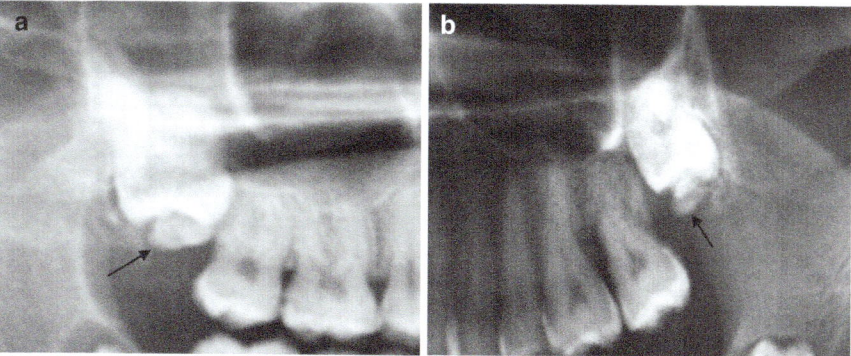

Fig. 7.16 (**a, b**) Two cases of dentinoma (indicated by *arrows*) in the occlusal surface of inclusive elements

Fig. 7.17 A case of complex odontoma (indicated by *arrows*)

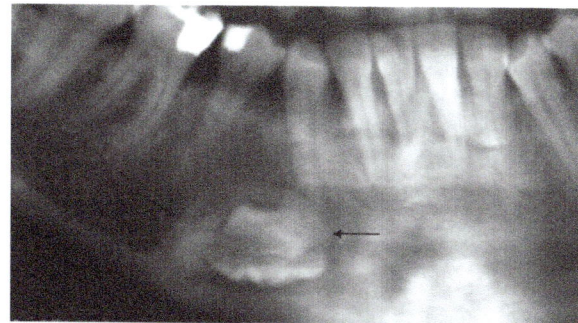

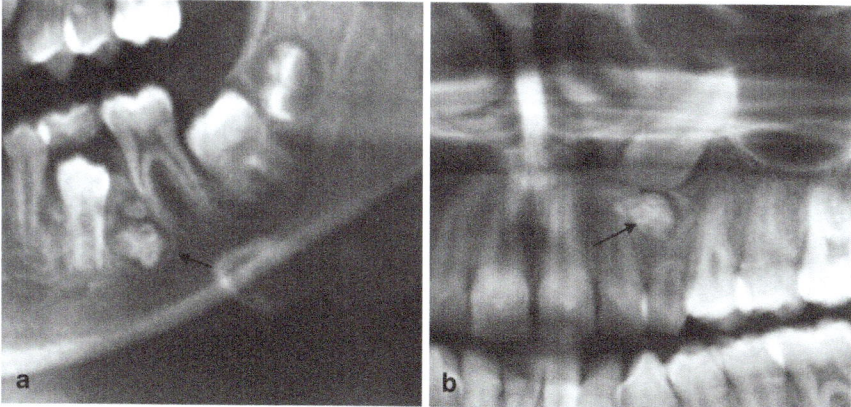

Fig. 7.18 (**a, b**) Two cases of compound odontoma. In (b) the finding is associated with the retention of the element 2.3 (see *arrows*)

Fig. 7.19 Adenomatoid odontogenic tumour constituted by a pericoronal cystic component (indicated by *short arrows*) and by a peripheral calcification (indicated by *long arrows*). The case has been erroneously considered as dentigerous cyst

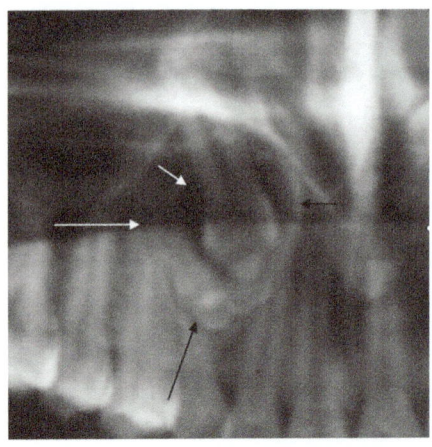

Fig. 7.20 Squamous odontogenic tumour. Osteolysis (indicated by *arrows*) centred on the apical region of 1.2, which is completely normal. The lesion has been erroneously considered as radicular cyst of 1.1

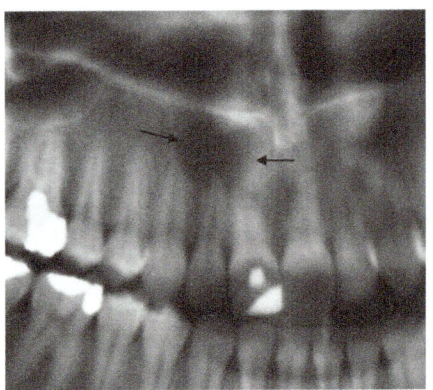

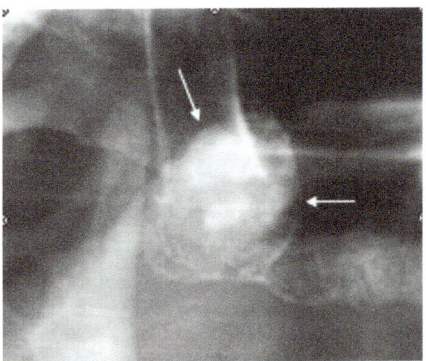

Fig. 7.21 Calcified formation developing in the sinusal cavity (indicated by *arrows*), erroneously interpreted as osteoma

Fig. 7.22 Monolocular ameloblastoma. Totally nonspecific finding of osteolysis with sharp outlines (indicated by *arrows*) of the angular region of the mandible

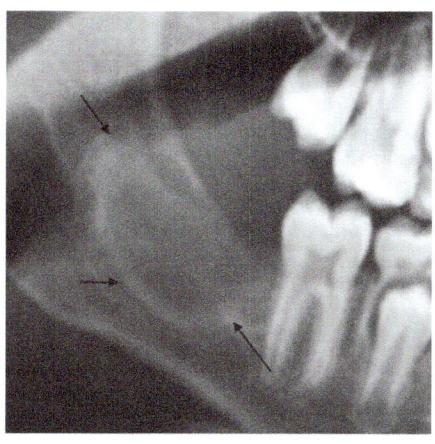

Fig. 7.23 Extended lytic lesion (ameloblastoma) erroneously interpreted as radicular cyst centred on 3.6. The *arrows* indicate the presence of a posterior component with multilocular aspect

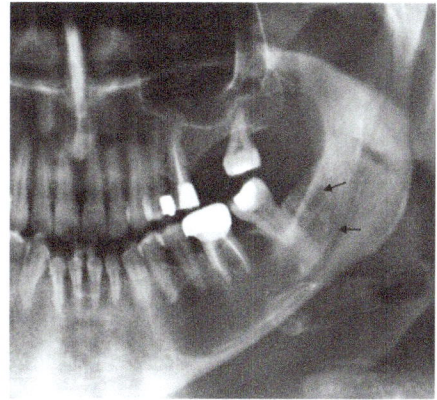

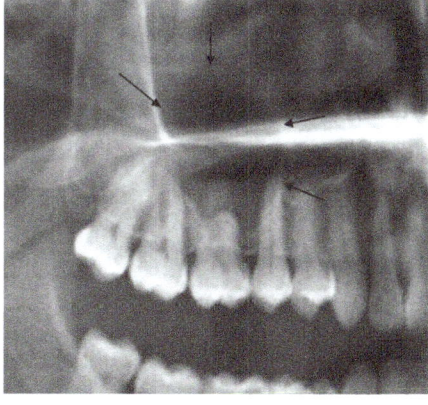

Fig. 7.24 Rare localisation of ameloblastoma in the right superior maxillary. The lesion (indicated by *arrows*) has been erroneously interpreted as radicular cyst for the alterations of the apices of 1.6

Fig. 7.25 Schematic diagram illustrating the seat of the two main median fissural cysts. (*1*) Cyst of the nasopalatine canal and (*2*) median fissural cyst. The *arrow* indicates the nasopalatine canal

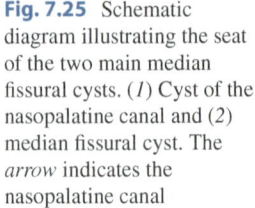
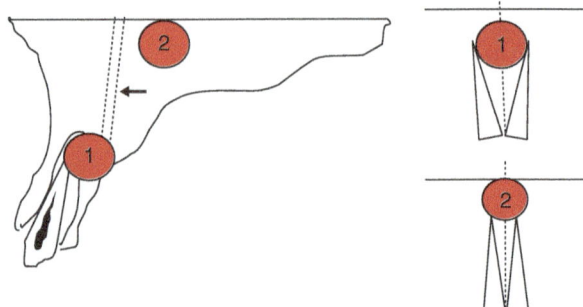

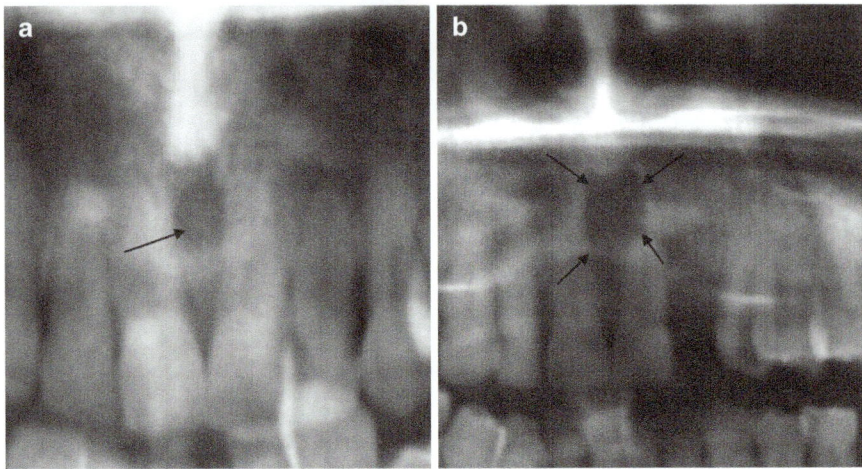

Fig. 7.26 (**a**) Cyst of the naso palatine canal (indicated by *arrow*). (**b**) Median fissural cyst (indicated by *arrows*). In the first one a slight diastasis of the median incisors is present

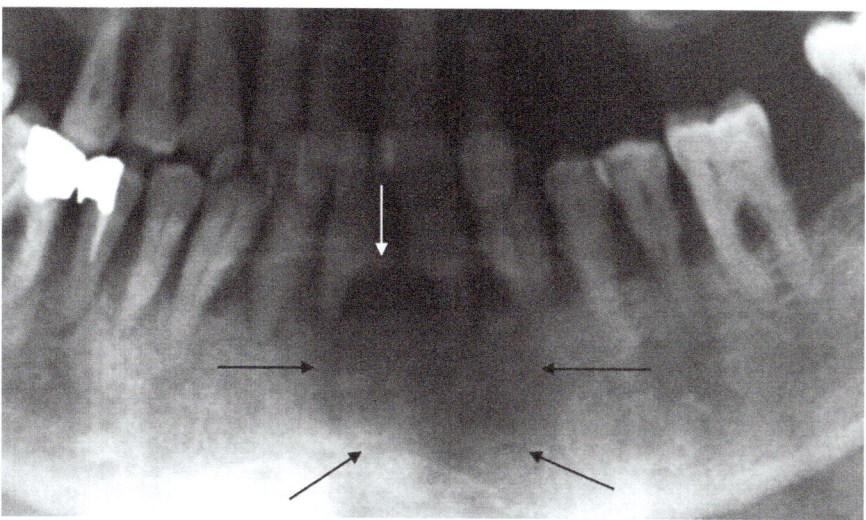

Fig. 7.27 Extended cystic lesion (indicated by *arrow*) of the region of the mental symphysis (occasional finding) which causes a certain instability of the central incisors

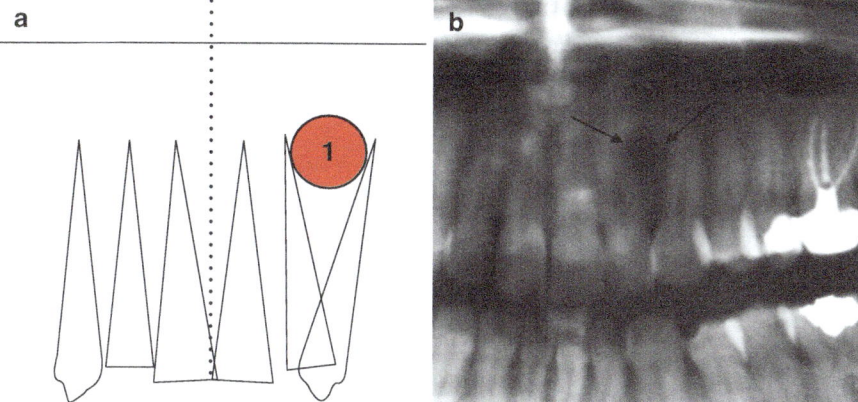

Fig. 7.28 Schematic representation (**a**) and radiographical representation (**b**) of globulomaxillary cyst (indicated by *arrows*)

Fig. 7.29 Wide osteolysis (indicated by *arrows*) due to carcinoma arising in the retromolar trigone with the involvement of the soft tissues. The distal root of 4.7 turns out to be included in the pathological tissue

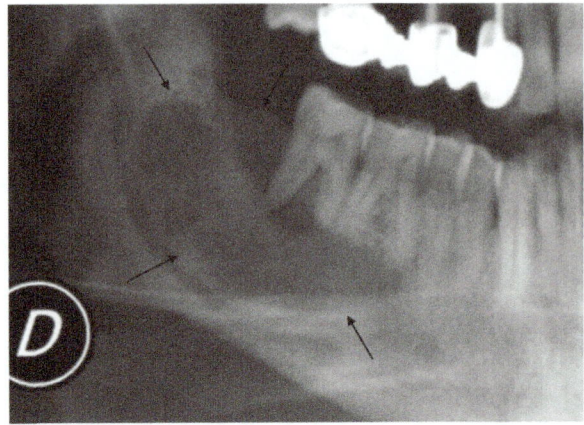

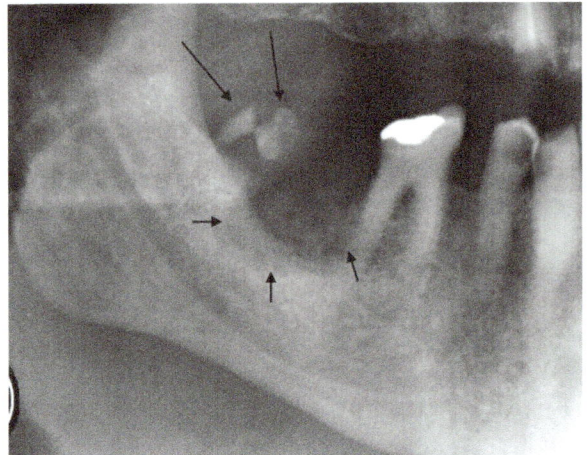

Fig. 7.30 Totally nonspecific osteolysis due to gingival carcinoma (indicated by *short arrows*). The *long arrows* indicate the dental residuals relocated by the soft component of the tumour

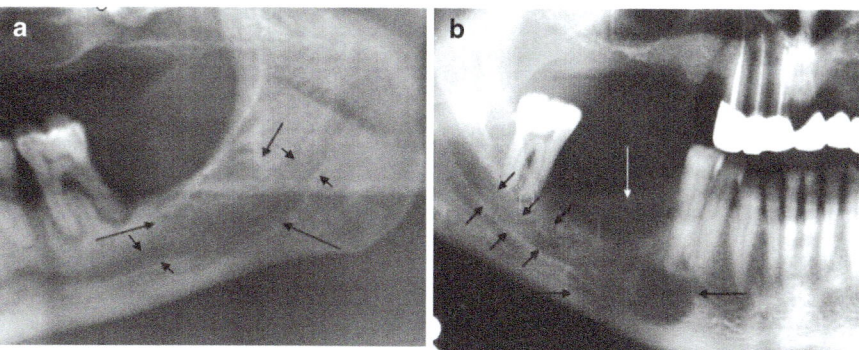

Fig. 7.31 (**a, b**) Two cases of mandibular osteolysis (indicated by *long arrows*) due to adenoid cystic carcinoma of the minor salivary glands of the oral cavity. This causes the widening of the mandibular canal (indicated by *short arrows*) due to perineural diffusion

Fig. 7.32 Schwannoma of the inferior alveolar nerve. Osteolysis with sharp outlines with geographical aspect (indicated by *arrows*), coaxial to the mandibular canal

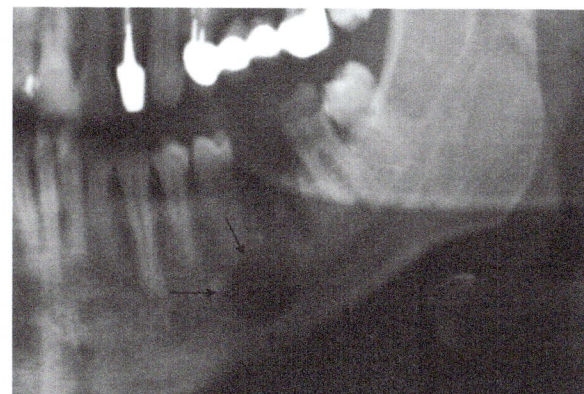

Fig. 7.33 Arteriovenous fistula expressed by the presence of osteolysis with sharp outlines with geographical aspect (indicated by *long arrow*). The mandibular canal turns out to be split (indicated by *short arrows*). Indeed, the superior canal constitutes the passage of the ectasic vascular axis characterised by an independent course with respect to the nerve which is contained in the canal located inferiorly

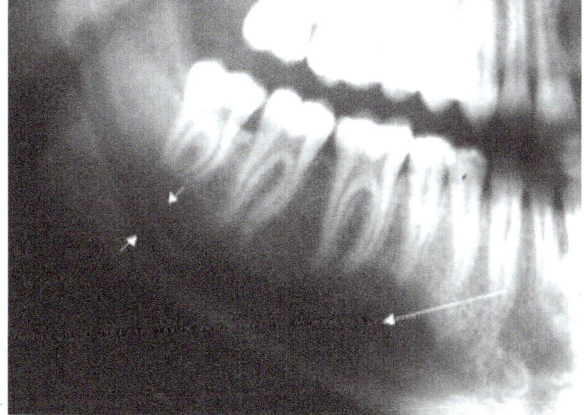

Suggested Reading

Adekeye EO (1980) Ameloblastoma of the jaws: a survey of 109 Nigerian patients. J Oral Surg 38:36–41

Allen CM et al (1998) Adenomatoid dentinoma. Report of four cases or an unusual odontogenic lesion. Oral Surg Oral Med Oral Pathol Oral Radiol Endod 86:313–317

Araki M, Matsumoto K, Matsumoto N, Honda K, Ohki H, Komiyama K (2010) Unusual radiographic appearance of ossifying fibroma in the left mandibular angle. Dentomaxillofac Radiol 39(5):314–319

Atkinson CH, Harwood AR, Cummings BJ (1984) Ameloblastoma of the jaw: a reappraisal of the role of irradiation. Cancer 53:869–873

Bodner L, Woldenberg Y, Bar-Ziv J (2003) Radiographic features of large cystic lesions of the jaws in children. Pediatr Radiol 33:3–6

Brannon RB (1976) The odontogenic keratocyst: a clinicopathologic study of 312 cases: I. Clinical features. Oral Surg Oral Med Oral Pathol 42:54–57

Brannon RB (1977) The odontogenic keratocyst: a clinicopathologic study of 312 cases: II. Histologic features. Oral Surg Oral Med Oral Pathol 42:233–255

Dahl E, Wolfson S, Haugen J (1981) Central odontogenic fibroma. J Oral Surg 39:120–124

Daley TD, Wysocki GP, Bringle GA (1994) Relative incidence of odontogenic tumors and oral jaw cyst in a Canadian population. Oral Surg Oral Med Oral Pathol Oral Radiol Endod 77:276–280

Dallera P, Bertoni F, Marchetti C et al (1994) Ameloblastoma fibrosarcoma of the jaw: report of five cases. J Craniomaxillofac Surg 77:276–280

Friedrich RE, Scheuer HA, Fuhrmann A, Zustin J, Assaf AT (2012) Radiographic findings of odontogenic myxomas on conventional radiographs. Anticancer Res 32(5):2173–2177

Gardner DG (1980) The central odontogenic fibroma: an attempt at clarification. Oral Surg Oral Med Oral Pathol 50:425–432

Gupta M, Kaste SC, Hopkins KP (2002) Radiologic appearance of primary jaw lesions in children. Pediatr Radiol 32:153–166

Ida M, Tetsumura A, Kuribayashi A, Okada N, Kurabayashi T (2012) A clinicoradiological study of odontogenic carcinomas and their impact on clinical diagnosis. Dentomaxillofac Radiol 41(7):594–600

Kerezoudis NP, Donta-Bakoyianni C, Siskos G (2000) The lateral periodontal cyst: aetiology, clinical significance and diagnosis. Endod Dent Traumatol 16(4):144–150

Kramer IRH, Pindborg JJ, Shear M (1992) Histologic typing of odontogenic tumours, 2nd edn, World Health Organization. Springer, Berlin/Heidelberg

Lovas J (1991) Cyst. In: Miles D, Van Dis M, Kangars G, Lovas J (eds) Oral and maxillofacial radiology. Radiologic/pathologic correlations. Saunders, Philadelphia

Mehkri S, Rajkumar GC, Nagesh KS, Manjunath GS (2012) Bilateral adenomatoid odontogenic tumour of the maxilla in a 2-year-old female–the report of a rare case and review of the literature. Dentomaxillofac Radiol 41(4):342–348

Philpsen HP et al (1999) Adenomatoid odontogenic tumor: facts and figures. Oral Oncol 35(2):125–131

Scholl RJ, Kellet HM, Neumann DP, Lurie AG (1999) Cysts and cystic lesions of the mandible: clinical and radiologic-histopathologic review. Radiographics 19:1107–1124

Shimamoto H, Kishino M, Okura M, Chindasombatjaroen J, Kakimoto N, Murakami S, Furukawa S (2011) Radiographic features of a patient with both cemento-ossifying fibroma and keratocystic odontogenic tumor in the mandible: a case report and review of literature. Oral Surg Oral Med Oral Pathol Oral Radiol Endod 112(6):798–802

Shimoyama T, Horie N, Nasu D et al (1999) So-called simple cyst of the jaw: a family of pseudocysts of diverse nature and etiology. J Oral Sci 41:93–98

OPT in Post-treatment Evaluation

8

General Considerations

There is no doubt that OPT is not the methodology of choice for the evaluation and checking of odontoiatric therapy results.

Indeed, this function is generally performed during the treatment through endoral radiograms and in case of sequela and/or major complications, through computed tomography.

However, it is true that the radiologist, while analysing an OPT radiogram, often has to face different treatment results and can have difficulty in making the report, especially if a precise query and/or a clinical recall are absent.

It must be said that the evaluation, based only on radiological findings, turns out to be very limited and sometimes misleading, if considered separately from the clinical context.

The aim of this chapter is to illustrate the main iconographic patterns related to the results of the different odontoiatric treatments as well as precising their issues and related terminology.

Radiological aspects related to **extractive therapy** and **conservative endodontic treatments** along with some of the issues related to **implantology** will be discussed.

Radiological Findings of the Extractive Treatments

Radiological findings related to the results of a previous **dental avulsion** mainly refer to the morphological analysis of the so-called extraction site.

It seems to be evident that radiological evaluation must always be supported by a minimum of clinical integration because the exclusive morphological interpretation can be misleading.

I. Pandolfo, S. Mazziotti, *Orthopantomography*,
DOI 10.1007/978-88-470-5289-5_8, © Springer-Verlag Italia 2013

Propaedeutical to the evaluation of the pathological extractive site is the knowledge of its normal morphology and its modifications occurring over time. The latter parameter is subjected to significant and very heterogeneous individual variations.

The main characteristic of a recent extraction site, in absence of pathological conditions, is the clear observation of all the anatomical components of the empty alveolus, which can be detectable for a variable time (30–40 days) from one subject to another.

Successively, the empty alveolus starts losing the sharpness of its outlines and assumes a blurred aspect. This is due to the proliferation and organisation of the granulation tissue, followed by mineralisation phenomena, which will lead in about 6–8 months to the complete bone obliteration of the alveolar cavity (Fig. 8.1a–c).

In some cases the blood clot, which is normally expected to occupy the extraction site, can be lost and the healing process interrupted or delayed.

The blood clot is, in fact, an important factor for the protection of the alveolar bone, and its loss can determine a painful complication called **alveolar osteitis** or **dry socket**.

In its early stage, obviously, such complication cannot be demonstrated through OPT.

The persistence of such pathological condition, generally linked to infection, determines the **subacute** and **chronic post-extractive alveolitis**.

As consequence the site can assume altered connotations which modify its characteristics. The main pathological modification comprises the reduction in sharpness of the alveolar cavity's outlines.

This finding (typical also of the site's normal evolution) has pathological meaning only if associated to the loss of the normal alveolar morphology.

Another significant element is represented by the diffuse osteosclerosis of the perialveolar cancellous bone, indicative of **sclerosing alveolitis** or **sclerosing osteitis** (Figs. 8.2a–c and 8.3).

Other factors concerning the radiological evaluation of an extraction site are related to a possible detection of **residual tooth fragments** or of **fracture lesions of the alveolar walls**.

Residual tooth fragments are found, most of the time, through endoral examinations during an extraction procedure, when the dentist suspects their presence. However, such a finding can occasionally be detected during OPT. In such cases, the clinical-anamnestic evaluation of the patient is obviously crucial for a correct interpretation of this radiological finding, which can often have little pathological significance (Fig. 8.4a, b).

Alveolar fractures are a consequence of extraction manoeuvres. When these lesions occur in the alveolar walls, on the vestibular or lingual-palatal sides, they cannot be detected by OPT for well-known projective reasons.

Conversely, it will be possible to give evidence of the possible lesions affecting the interradicular crest, whose fragment can sometimes contribute to phenomena of post-extractive alveolitis. The fragment can assume the aspect of a small osteosclerotic sequestration inside the alveolus (Fig. 8.5a, b).

Moreover, the radiological analysis of the extraction site must consider possible damages in the mandibular canal, or in the floor of the maxillary sinus, with the consequent formation of **oroantral fistula** (Figs. 8.6a, b and 8.7).

One must consider that during its evolution, the extraction site may not have its normal bone obliteration. This is most likely to happen for reasons related to chronic inflammatory phenomena, which are often oligosymptomatic.

In this eventuality, the extraction site will develop into an irreversible residual cavity, characterised by little clinical relevance.

In order to prevent this unfavourable situation, some dentists accumulate radiopaque and resorbable material in the post-extraction cavity (Fig. 8.8a, b).

Finally, the possibility for the extraction site to be in continuity with the small residual cavity due to the apical granuloma must be taken in account (Fig. 8.9).

Effects of the Endodontic Therapy

This **conservative therapy**, aiming at saving the dental element, is fundamentally based on the techniques of **endodontic treatment** which consider penetrating caries, with infection of the dental pulp (**pulpitis**), to be the main indication.

The treatment consists of eliminating the carious lesion as well as the removal of the altered pulp from the pulp chamber and canals (**devitalisation**), followed by obliteration of pulp chamber and canals, through radiopaque resin-based material (**gutta-percha**), in order to seal the aforementioned cavities. This last procedure avoids persistence and/or diffusion of the infection (**canalar therapy**).

It is clear that all the aforesaid procedure can be evaluated by the dentist while operating, through the use of endoral radiograms.

In the evaluation of a panoramic radiogram, the morphological results of these procedures are often evident. Moreover, their analysis cannot be prescinded from a clinical-anamnestic evaluation.

Indeed, also in the presence of extremely insufficient results on the morphological aspect, it is not rare to notice clinical conditions which are totally normal and vice versa.

The main problems that must be considered in the presence of the canalar therapy results are irregular and **incomplete canal filling, endocanalar overfilling** and **false routes**.

The aforementioned evaluations obviously presume familiarity with a perfect realised treatment. In particular the filling must reproduce the morphology of the pulp chamber and of one or more canals (**endodontic cone**) in complete manner, without any irregularities or discontinuities (Fig. 8.10a–c).

Irregular and Incomplete Canal Filling

The finding of irregular, discontinuous and incomplete canal filling seems to contradict the rationale on which endodontic treatment is based.

Indeed, segments of the pulp-canal cavity which have not been obliterated by the radiopaque material cause a risk of microbial persistence and proliferation in this area.

However, it must be said that in presence of these morphological pictures, the radiological evaluation must be subordinated to the clinical one.

The existence of a periapical lesion indicates the inadequacy of this treatment (Fig. 8.11a–c).

Sometimes, periapical lesions can be detectable even in the presence of endodontic treatments which are morphologically impeccable (Fig. 8.12).

In this case, they can be considered either a vestigial remain of a periapical lesion now eradicated and destined to bone obliteration or a conspicuous inflammatory lesion in evolution.

Apart from the clinical evaluation, the only criterion (although quite unpredictable) able to distinguish between two hypothesis is its evolution by the time.

As a matter of fact, vestigial lesions tend to disappear within the space of 3–4 years.

Similar considerations are related to the results of the surgical treatment through **apicectomy**.

Indeed, this therapeutic method entails the resection of the root tip of the tooth (previous **microsurgical transgingival approach**) and of the periapical lesion. This has to be obviously preceded by the endodontic treatment of the pulp chamber and the radicular canal.

In these cases, as remains of the surgical treatment, a lytic lesion adjacent to the resected apex can be detected. Such lesion, if therapeutic success occurs, will be obliterated as time goes by (Fig. 8.13).

The **restoration of the crown** completes the endodontic treatment.

This procedure can be realised with different techniques which see the employment of materials characterised by variable (from modest to marked) opacity.

The use of materials characterised by modest opacity or one which is otherwise inferior to that of the normal elements' crown must not generate the erroneous interpretation of carious lesion (Fig. 8.14).

The crown restoration device often becomes integral with the radicular complex through the insertion of a metallic post (**endodontic post**) (Fig. 8.15a, b).

The endodontic post can also be associated to alterations of the adjacent dental tissue through resorption phenomena. On the clinical point of view, this event can be similar to those caused by situations related to insufficient or incomplete canal filling and, in addition, to more or less significant dental instability (Fig. 8.16).

Overfilling of the Radicular Canal

The canal filling is considered as excessive when the radiopaque material, exceeding the apical foramen, spreads inside the surrounding periapical tissues.

This condition, within certain limits, does not have any pathological significance (Fig. 8.17a–c) even though sometimes, most likely related to chemical reaction or bacterial contamination, clinical and radiological signs of osteitis can appear (Fig. 8.18).

Of major clinical relevance is the outflow of the filling material towards critical anatomical structures such as the mandibular canal or the floor of the maxillary sinus, whose mucosa turns out to be particularly vulnerable to chemical and/or mechanical stimuli produced by the aforementioned material (Fig. 8.19).

False Routes

During an endodontic treatment, because of incongruous manoeuvres and/or in the presence of altered or however complex anatomical situations, a breach into an erroneous anatomical area can occur. As a consequence, the filling material will be introduced outside the limits of the canal cavity.

The negative consequences of such an event are twofold: on one hand the cleaning of the canal will be missed, and on the other hand filling material which is introduced outside the tooth may cause damages into the surrounding tissues

The latter eventuality is particularly significant when the erroneous course causes the involvement of the periodontal space (Fig. 8.20).

In OPT, the observation of erroneous courses is not a frequent event as, in the majority of cases, the problem is detected or at least suspected during treatment and therefore documented through endoral radiograms. As a consequence, the error is almost always eliminated.

Extravasations outside the dental limits due to false routes can be an occasional finding during OPT, especially when the phenomenon has passed unnoticed for its poor clinical relevance (Fig. 8.21a, b).

OPT in the Postimplantation Evaluation

In the preimplantation phase, OPT, which is a methodology of first level, is able to acquire complex and general information concerning the masticatory apparatus. Such data are useful both in the view of the implantation strategy planning and for the legal-medical aims in order to provide documentary evidence of the pretreatment condition of the patient.

OPT allows us to furnish a judgement on the presence and extension of **periodontal disease**, possible inflammatory lesions, **retained elements**, **radicular remains**, etc.

These evaluations alone, though very useful, are not able to support correct preimplantation planning. This is due to the fact that some parameters, such as the thickness of the alveolar bone, the inclination of the alveolar ridges and the directional and topographic rapports of the implantation device with the anatomical structures of reference, are not reliably detected in OPT. This is related to the impossibility of tridimensional evaluations and the distortion generated by geometric radiographic enlargement.

It follows that a correct preimplantation planning must be set taking into account the more complex methodologies of second level, such as computed tomography (through **Dentascan** technique)and **cone beam**.

OPT only plays a supporting role even during the intraoperative phase. This occurs in the presence of particular anatomical situations, in which the correct positioning of an implantation device cannot be adequately evaluated through endoral examination.

In the final evaluation of the treatment, OPT provides the definitive and global documentation, which is useful as temporal reference for eventual further controls and/or interventions.

In order to evaluate possible failures and/or major complications, besides the possible legal-medical dispute, OPT turns out to be ancillary to the methodologies of second level.

It is clear that OPT is not a methodology able to conclusively evaluate the results of an implantation treatment, but is often able to provide judgement of relevant elements.

On this basis, the radiologist must be aware of the main issues subtended by a treatment, besides having knowledge of the materials and their relative terminology.

Topographic Subdivision of the Maxillary in Implantation Perspective

In implantology both the superior and the inferior maxillaries are topographically subdivided into zones or sectors, each of which is characterised by peculiarity which make it more or less suitable and critical with respect to the procedure.

Figures 8.22 and 8.23 schematically illustrate these zone or sectors, with their relative nomenclature.

It is evident that, for example, the sector of the **canine pillar**, because of its remarkable thickness, will be more appropriate for the positioning of longer implantation devices and therefore potentially more stable.

Conversely, the **subantral sector** appears critical both for the frequent modest thickness of the alveolar bone and for the rapports with the overhanging maxillary sinus.

The **maxillary tuberosity sector** represents a potential implantation seat, in order to obviate a serious deficiency of the bone of the subantral region.

However, this area presents more relevant technical difficulties due to the presence of the **pterygoid process** and the **pterygopalatine fossa**, as well as the **palatine artery** and the **palatine nerve**.

In the inferior maxillary, the most critical areas are mainly characterised by the **periforaminal sector** and the **posterior sector** for the possible rapports between the implantation devices and the inferior alveolar nerve.

Different Typologies of Implantation Devices

In the last years, advances in implantology have been strictly linked to technological evolution. This has seen the introduction of more intuitive implantation devices (or **fixtures**), based on scientifically incontrovertible physical and biomechanical criteria.

In a quite short time, obsolete devices now rarely in use, such as **blade** or **pin implants**, have been replaced by numerous types of **screw implants** which offer a wide range of models (Figs. 8.24 and 8.25a–d).

The most state-of-the-art implants, now more frequently employed, have been designed in order to make the devices more similar to the morphology of a tooth.

To fulfil this aim, a series of devices, constituted by a single stem (which reproduces the radicular axis of the tooth) equipped with a spiral screw and a neck, have been generated.

Implant dimensions (length and calliper) are chosen depending on the anatomical characteristics of the implant site.

The most used implants are hollow along their whole length to provide a seat (sealed by an apposite **closure screw**), in which a metal **pillar** (**abutment**) is inserted. This is characterised by different morphology and angulations, depending on how the definitive crown prosthesis is anchored on the implant (Figs. 8.26, 8.27a, b and 8.28).

This technique is called **biphasic implant procedure**, as between the positioning of the implant device and the pillar insertion (abutment) some time is needed (4–6 months) in order to integrate the implant stem with the alveolar bone.

During this time, the implant, sealed by the closure screw, can be free or covered by the gingiva.

Obviously, in this last eventuality, the abutment positioning must foresee the incision of the gingival plane and the application of a further screw (known as **healing screw**) which aims at remodelling the gingival plane.

The aforementioned implants, in addition to installing a crown device, can be employed to build the pillars of a bridge or to anchor a mobile dental prosthesis. For the latter aim, abutments with spherical endings (**ball abutments**) are used (Fig. 8.29).

Though the biphasic technique is the most employed in clinical practice, today the use of **monophasic implant technique** or **immediate load implant** is more and more widespread.

This methodology consists of the application of the implant, already equipped with connection pillar and crown prosthesis with immediate functional load. Therefore, it presents the benefit of being a treatment with highly reduced duration and costs (Fig. 8.30).

However, it must be underlined that the success of monophasic treatment mainly depends on accurate selection of patients whose most important requisite is a good **primary stability**, guaranteed by the quality of the receiving bone and the optimal biomechanical conditions.

Osseous Integration

Independently from the technique employed, the aim is to obtain the implant's maximum stability and duration through the achievement of complete **osseous integration**.

Osseous integration is a biological process which consists of the complete and long-lasting firm adherence of the bone tissue to the foreign body represented by the implant.

This process, which is at the basis of the implant procedure, is realised through the use of pure **titanium**, which is the constituent of the device.

Indeed, titanium is a biologically complete inert material and therefore is not able to cause inflammatory reactions or immunological phenomena which can invalidate the results of the procedure.

Consequently, it is believed that the majority of failures ending with instability of the implant device are caused either by pathological mechanical stress of a wrongly placed and angulated implant or by a failure to respect the selection criteria, which are related to bone structural conditions, patient's health and age, smoke habit, poor oral hygiene, etc.

These circumstances give rise to the concept of missing '**primary stability**', the most important cause of the implant procedure's failure.

Osseous integration is also fostered by roughening the surface of the implant; conversely, the surface of the neck turns out to be smooth.

The presence of the spiral screw also has the effect of promoting osseous integration, increasing the contact surface between bone and implant.

Osseous integration is mainly evaluated clinically, even if radiological examination can provide elements in order to formulate a judgement.

However, radiological findings integrate the clinical judgement providing very precise anatomical references which often allow a more accurate quantification of the damage.

The main pathological substrate of the missing integration is peri-implant bone resorption, event defined as **peri-implantitis**.

In truth, the use of this term is not always justified, as the bone resorption, at least in its initial phases, can recognise mechanical causes. Instead, inflammatory alterations usually appear later and are typical of instability situations characterised by major seriousness.

However, the radiological approach to this field must be supported by some basic knowledge, propaedeutical in order to achieve a correct evaluation.

Firstly, it must be precised that a modest bone resorption with cone morphology, typically localised in the region of the implant neck (area characterised by major mechanical stress), represents, especially in the first year, a normal event. Therefore, it must not be mentioned in the report (Fig. 8.31a, b).

Another criterion is based on the evaluation of the ratio between the length of the part of the implant emerging from the bone and its intraosseous part (**crown/root ratio**).

In optimal conditions, this ratio is characterised by the major length of the intraosseous component of the implant or, at most, by equal length between the two components (Fig. 8.32).

The cases, in which this relation tends to be reversed (because of the bone resorption along the implant's root), will be characterised by a more or less serious or, at least, potential condition of missing integration (Fig. 8.33a, b).

The **peri-implant bone resorption** can present itself in very variable ways.

Sometimes the radiological signs can be so modest that the radiological evaluation must be supported and guided by clinical judgement. Conversely if the alterations are more evident, the radiological interpretation will be easier (Fig. 8.34a, b).

In OPT evaluation carried out by digital technique, the possibility to overestimate the process of peri-implant demineralisation must be considered when processing algorithms generating a too strong edge enhancement effect are employed.

These reconstruction filters, in fact, can generate a typical artefact (**Uberschwinger** or **rebound artefact**), consisting in a halation of radiolucency, miming a resorption process at the interface level between bone and implant.

Consequently, optimal evidence of peri-implant bone conditions requires the use of reconstruction algorithms with more balanced reconstruction filters (Fig. 8.35a, b).

The extreme manifestations of missing osseous integration generate conditions of instability with significant change of position of the implants which are easily detected both by clinical and OPT evaluation (Figs. 8.36 and 8.37a–c).

The most critical anatomical structures, from the implantological point of view, are represented by the maxillary sinus, for what concerns the superior arcade, and by the inferior alveolar nerve in the inferior maxillary.

The maxillary sinus, as a consequence of the extreme fragility of the cancellous bone which constitutes the alveolar process in the subantral region, is often the seat of issues which are able to negatively affect the integration process of the implant.

In this perspective, it is possible that the apex implant penetrating the cortical and the periosteum (**Schneider membrane**) comes into contact with the endosinusal area, causing inflammatory phenomena which are able to impede the success of the procedure.

The bidimensional radiological evaluation of such event through OPT is not easy, as the projective superimposition of the implant device and the maxillary sinus can prevent the demonstration of the very thin osteo-periosteal wall.

The only radiological criterion able to detect the presence of the sinus wall perforation is related to the evidence provided by the signs of sinus inflammation. These are the opacification of the cavity and/or the reactive thickening of the mucosa which is adjacent to the implant apex (Figs. 8.38 and 8.39).

The typical expression of the wall perforation is represented by the complete mobilisation and endosinusal displacement of the implant. This event is often caused both by the extreme thinness and fragility of the spongiosa of the alveolar ridge and by incongruous manoeuvres (Fig. 8.40a, b).

The evaluation of possible damage to the inferior alveolar nerve, caused by pathological contact between the implant apex and the nerve, is of major difficulty.

Indeed, the bidimensionality of the OPT image does not permit to distinguish between the simple projective superimposition and the real contact between the two structures (Fig. 8.41).

Therefore, it is obvious that this evaluation must be based only on an accurate clinical recall, and in its absence, radiological examination must not be considered as definitive.

Conversely, OPT turns out to be useful and efficient in the detection of the implant fractures (generally due to incongruous manoeuvres in the presence of implants characterised by unfavourable positioning and mechanical load conditions). Moreover, OPT detects the presence of implant fragments which are dispersed and retained in the maxillaries. Their existence is often ignored even by the patient (Figs. 8.42 and 8.43a, b).

These metal fragments, as known, can cause problems when it is necessary to plan further implant procedures or particular therapies, such as the somministration of drugs based on diphosphonates, or radiotherapeutic treatments.

To conclude this chapter, it is necessary to mention the possibility for OPT to evaluate the results related to a previous intervention of maxillary **sinus floor augmentation** also known as **sinus lift**.

This is a procedure aiming at increasing the subantral alveolar bone which makes possible the successive positioning of one or more implants.

The procedure consists of creating a surgical breach at the level of the alveolar bone followed by the detachment and lift of the periosteal membrane inside the maxillary sinus (**Schneider membrane**). It follows the introduction into the regained space of either the **autolog bone** (taken from the mandibular symphysis or the mandibular angle of the patient), opportunely particulated, or synthetic material.

After a certain amount of time, following the germination of the aforementioned material and the bone reconstruction, this technique will give rise to the appearance of a plaque with osteomatous-like opacity in which thickness an implant can be inserted (Fig. 8.44).

Obviously, the evaluation of the procedure's success is above all clinical. However, it seems to be appropriate and necessary for the radiologist to be aware of this technique and its possible complication as follows: infection, oroantral fistulas, sinusitis and tilting or loosening of implants.

Image Gallery

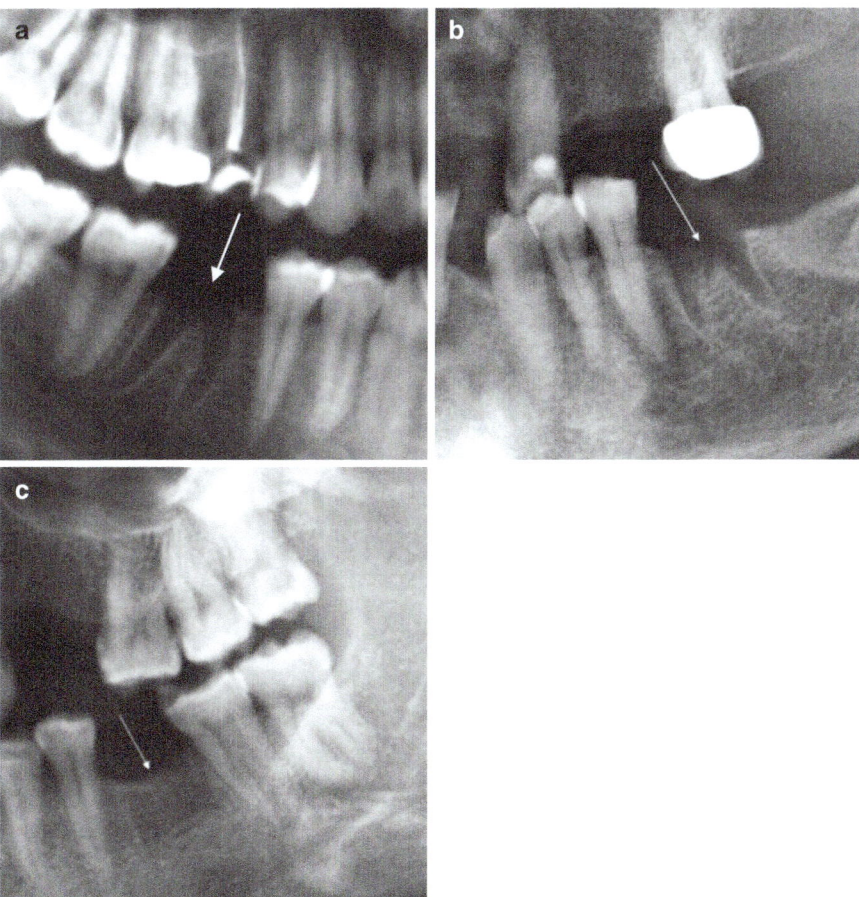

Fig. 8.1 Normal extraction sites (indicated by *arrows*). (**a**) Extraction site after 3 days. (**b**) Extraction site after 1 month. (**c**) Extraction site after 1 year. In (a, b) all the alveolar components are evident. In (b) the outlines start to lose their sharpness. In (c) the bone obliteration of the alveolar cavity is almost complete

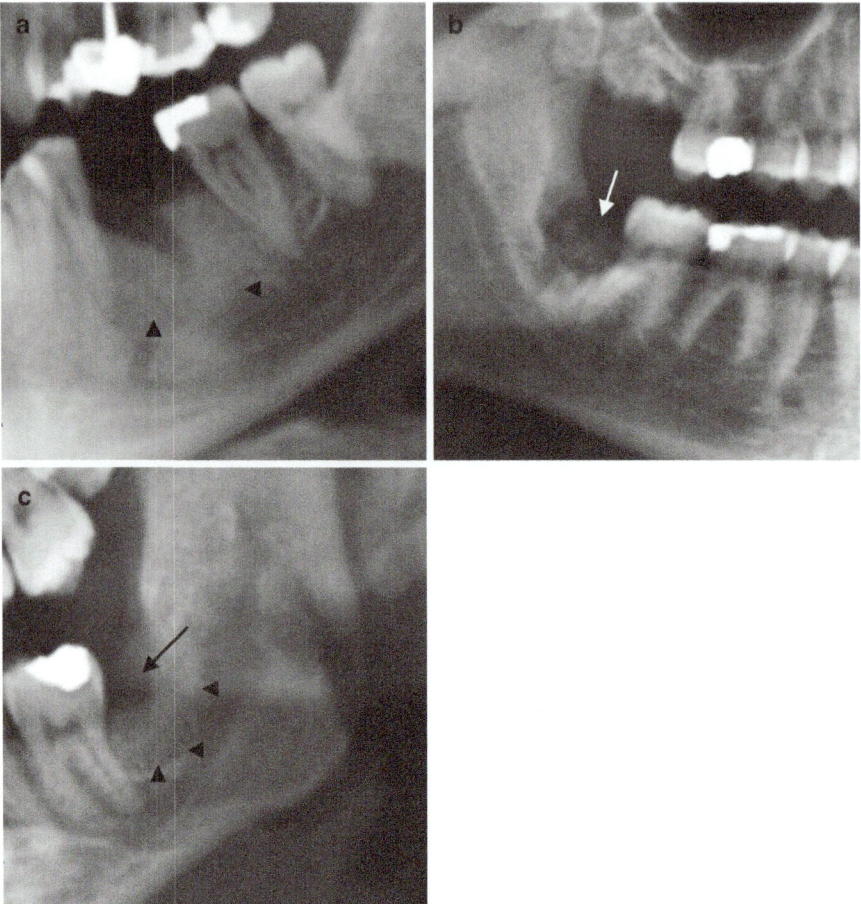

Fig. 8.2 Three situations of post-extraction alveolitis. In (**a**) alveolar morphology is maintained (indicated by *arrow*), and sclerosis of the spongiosa due to sclerosing osteitis is observable (*arrowheads*). In (**b**) alveolar morphology is altered (indicated by *arrow*). In (**c**) alveolar morphology is totally modified. A focal osteolysis is observable (indicated by *arrow*). This is due to the abscessual collection surrounded by bony sclerosis (indicated by *arrowheads*)

Fig. 8.3 The image shows three extraction sites in different evolution. The site in position 3.5 is the oldest and appears to be approaching bone obliteration. Site 3.6 is the most recent and appears to be normal. Site 3.7 presents blurred outlines and is surrounded by sclerosis ring (indicated by *arrows*). Both signs are indicative of post-extractive osteitis

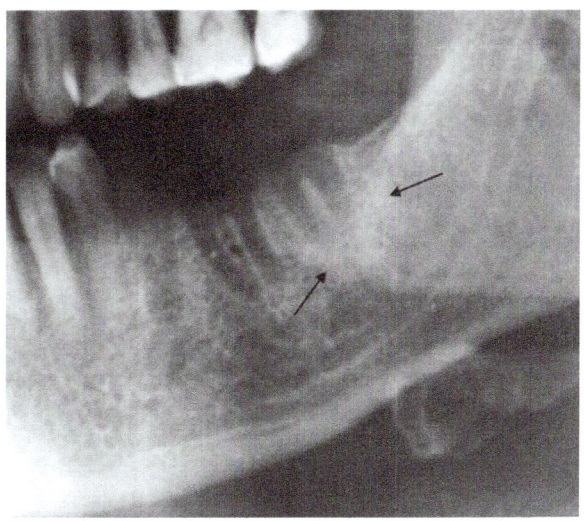

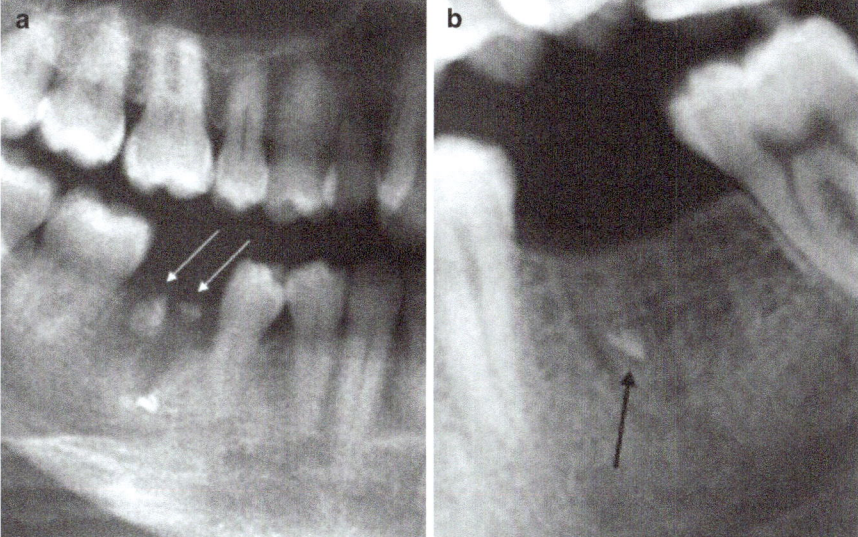

Fig. 8.4 (**a**) Dental fragments (indicated by *arrows*) in a recent extraction site. (**b**) Dental fragment (indicated by *arrow*) in an extraction site approaching bone obliteration. The finding does not have pathological significance

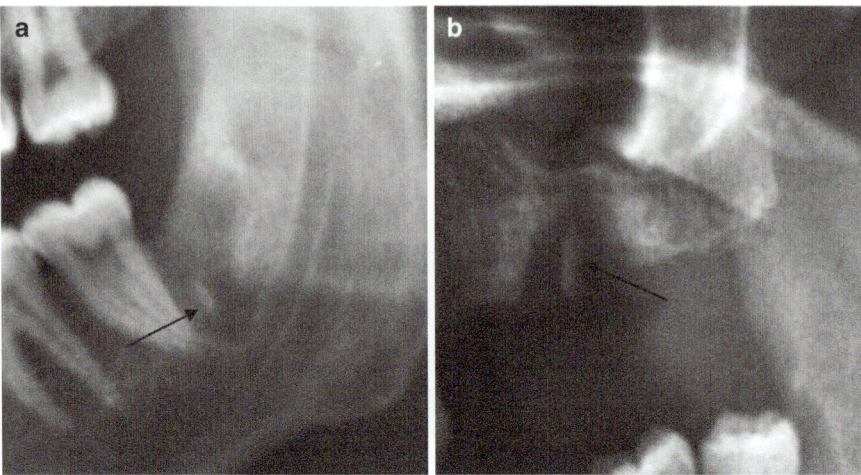

Fig. 8.5 In (**a**) a thin fractured fragment of the interradicular crest occurs (indicated by *arrow*). In (**b**) signs of chronic post-extraction alveolysis are present. The bony fragment (indicated by *arrow*) is sclerotic

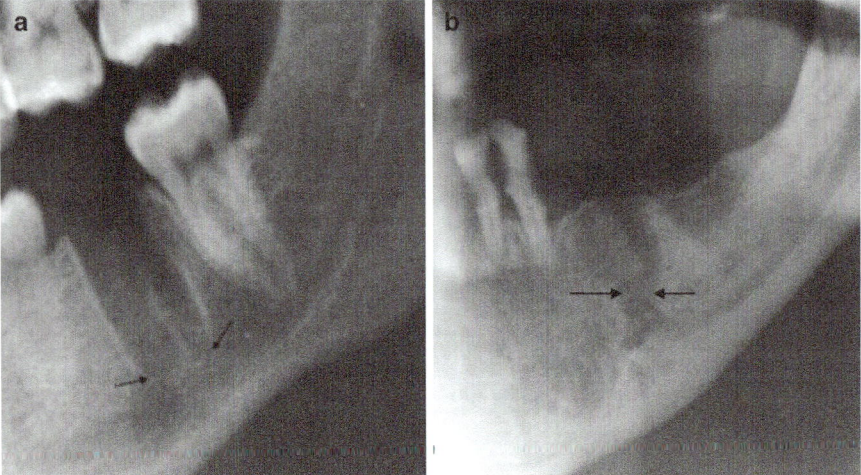

Fig. 8.6 In (**a**) disappearance of the cortical of the apical region (indicated by *arrows*). Hypotheses about the damage to the mandibular canal can be made. In (**b**) fistulous communication (indicated by *arrows*) between extraction site and mandibular canal is present

Fig. 8.7 Extraction site (indicated by *arrow*) communicating with the maxillary sinus

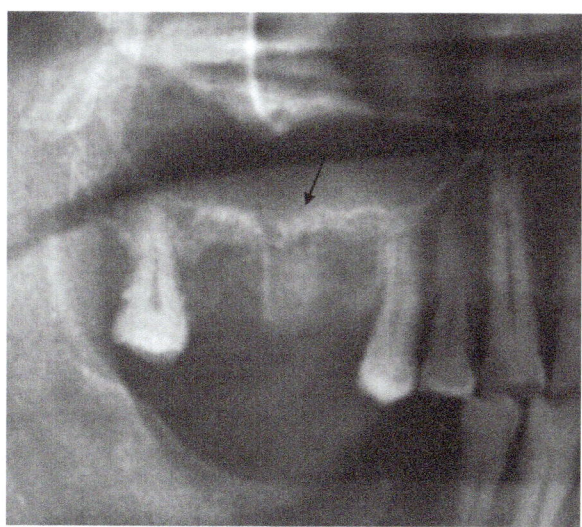

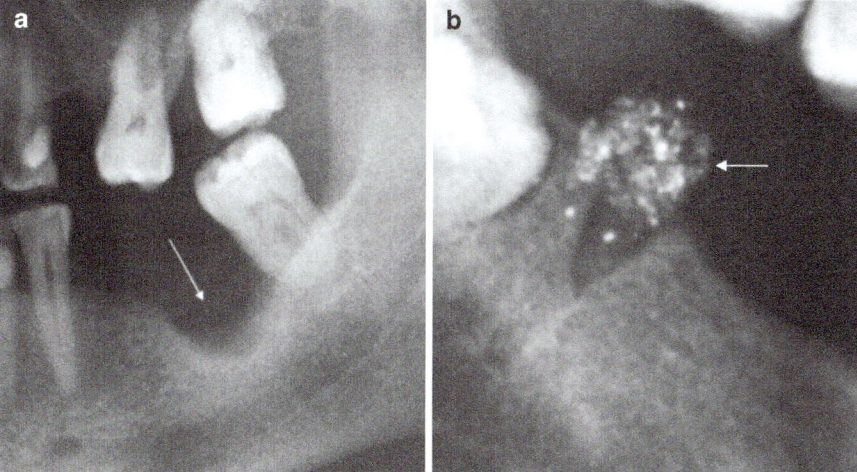

Fig. 8.8 (**a**) Extraction site evolved in residual cavity (indicated by *arrow*). (**b**) Extraction site with resorbable radiopaque material (indicated by *arrow*)

Fig. 8.9 Extraction site communicating with the cavity due to apical granuloma of the mesial root (indicated by *arrows*)

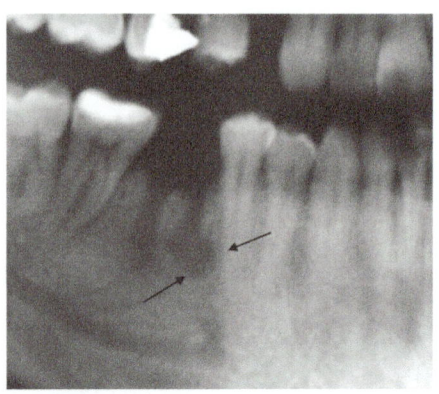

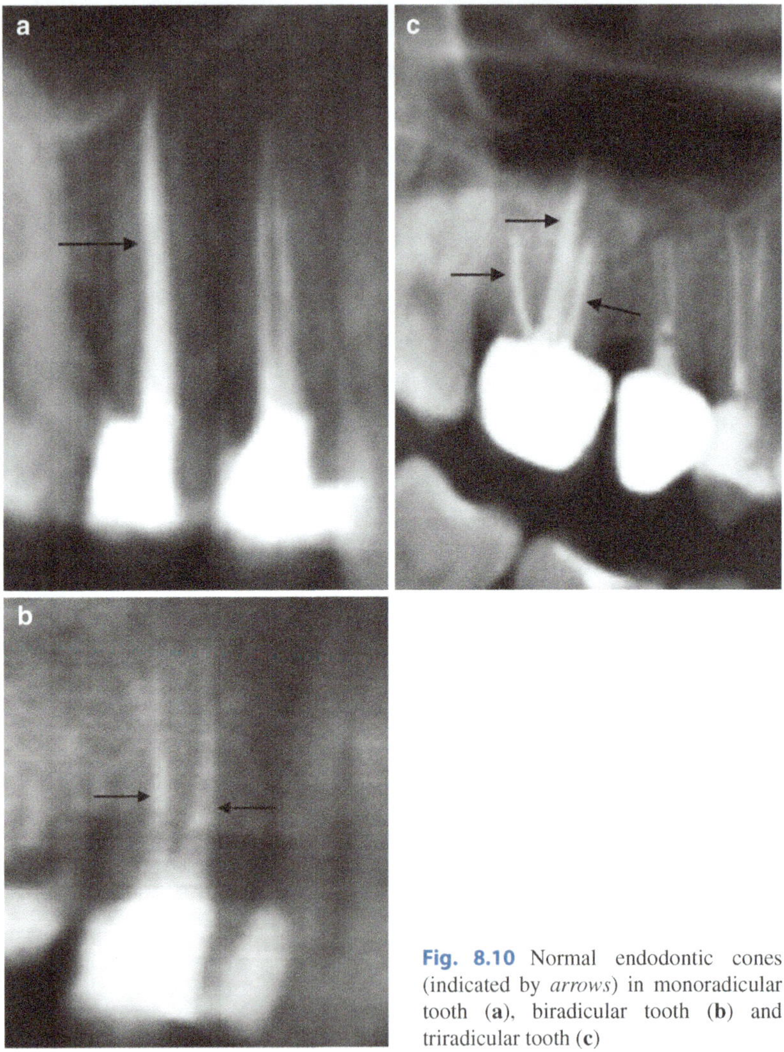

Fig. 8.10 Normal endodontic cones (indicated by *arrows*) in monoradicular tooth (**a**), biradicular tooth (**b**) and triradicular tooth (**c**)

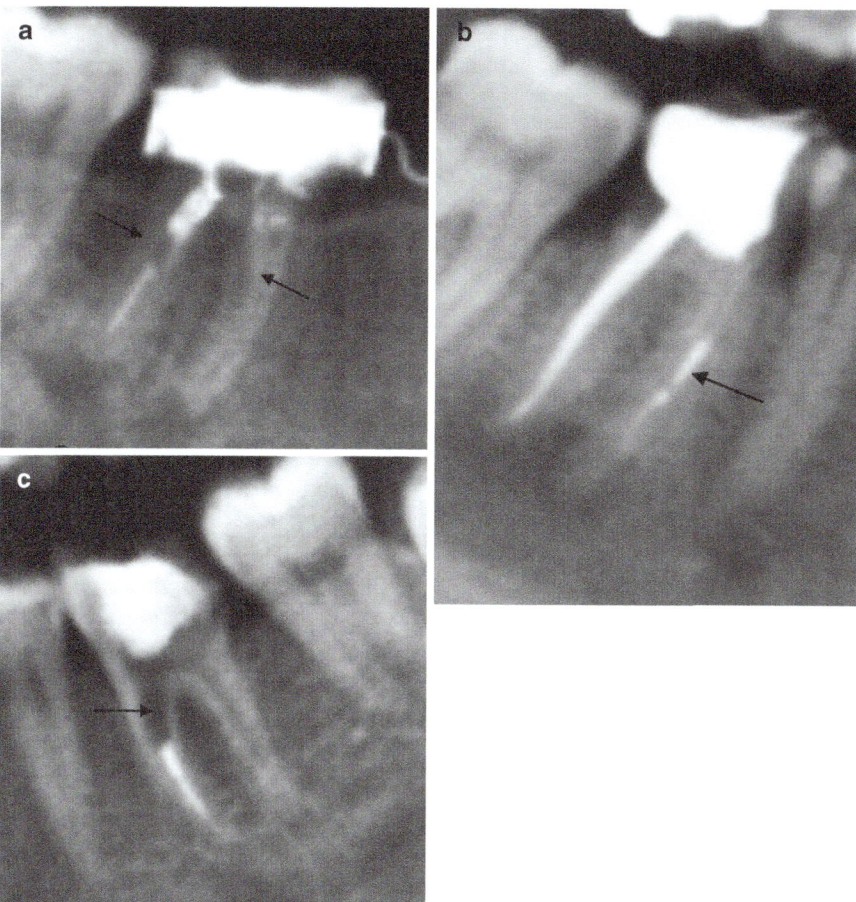

Fig. 8.11 Three examples of incomplete and irregular canal filling. In (**a**, **b**) periapical lesions are also present. In (**c**) widening of the radicular canal (indicated by *arrow*) due to endodontic damage is observable

Fig. 8.12 Periapical lesion (indicated by *arrow*) in a tooth with endodontic cone which is absolutely normal. Only clinical examination and its evolution are able to define the significance of the radiographic image

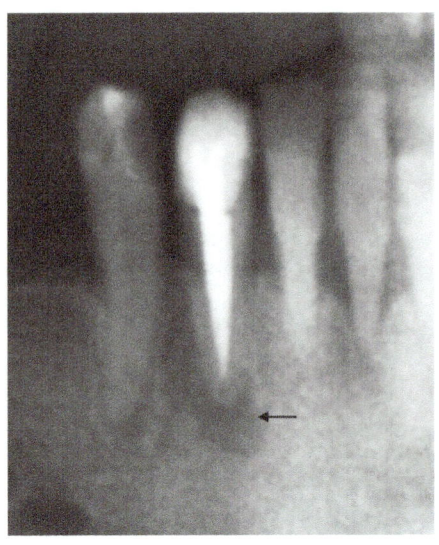

Fig. 8.13 Results of apicectomy (indicated by *short arrows*) with the presence of periapical residual demineralisation (indicated by *long arrows*)

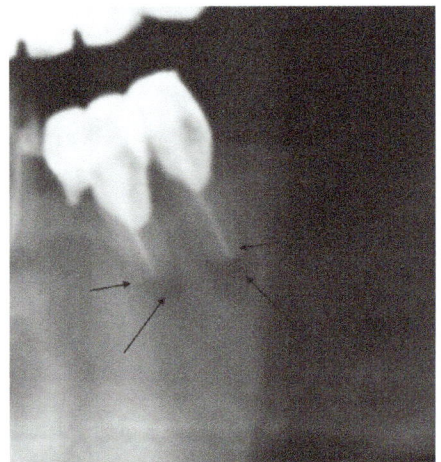

Fig. 8.14 Canalar therapy and coronal restoration with low-opacity material (indicated by *arrow*). This finding must not be confused with a carious lesion of the crown

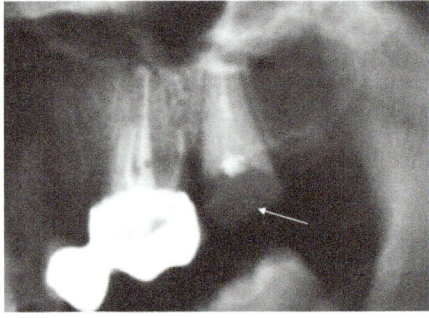

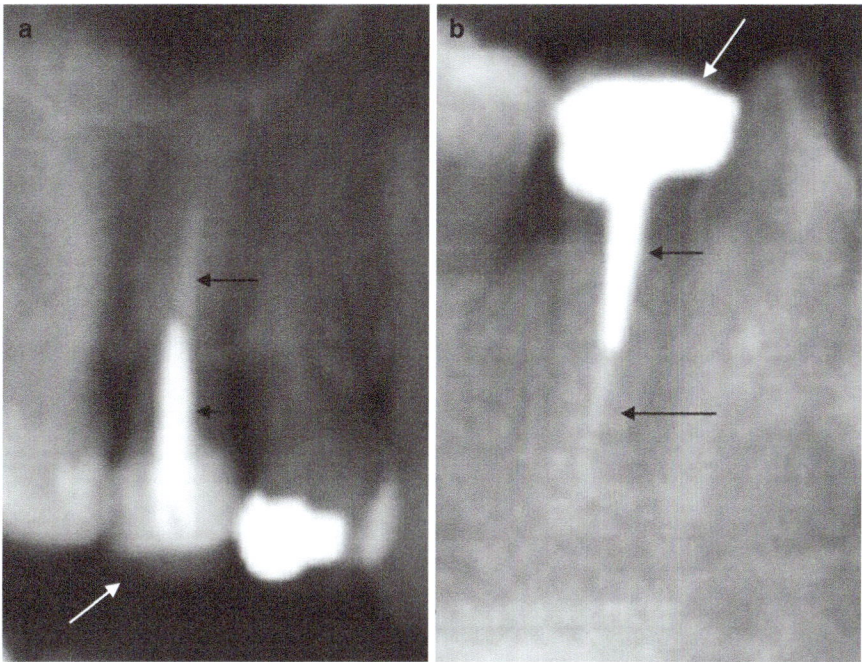

Fig. 8.15 Coronal restoration through endodontic post (indicated by *short arrows*) and canal obliteration (indicated by *long arrows*). In (**a**) the crown has been restored with less radiopaque material than in (**b**) (indicated by *white arrows*)

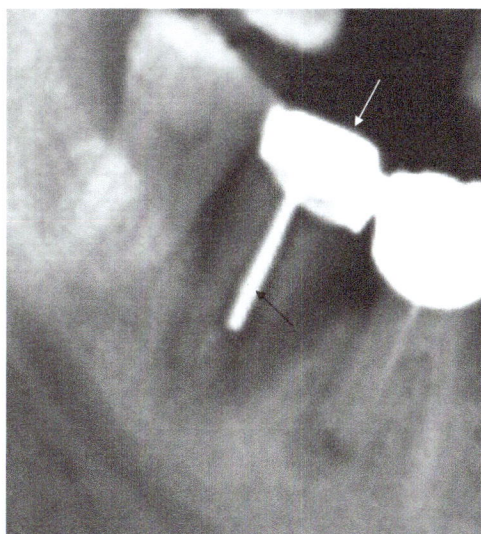

Fig. 8.16 Coronal device (indicated by *white arrow*) anchored through endodontic post (indicated by *black arrow*). It is unstable because of the resorption of the adjacent dentine

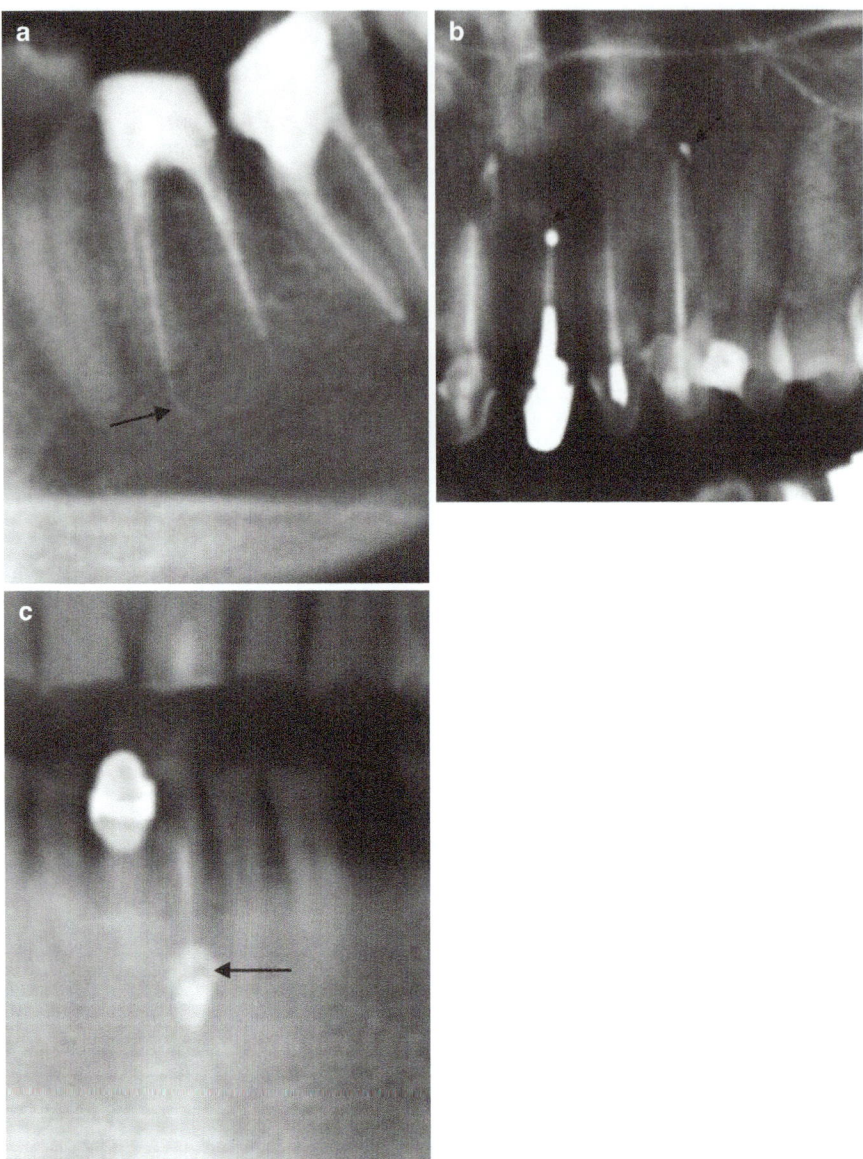

Fig. 8.17 (**a–c**) Three cases of overfilling with spread of modest quantities of gutta-percha (indicated by *arrows*) in the periapical area. The finding is very limited and has poor clinical relevance

Fig. 8.18 Overflow of the radiopaque material into the periapical area. Sclerosis of the spongiosa (indicated by *arrows*) is due to the presence of inflammatory phenomena

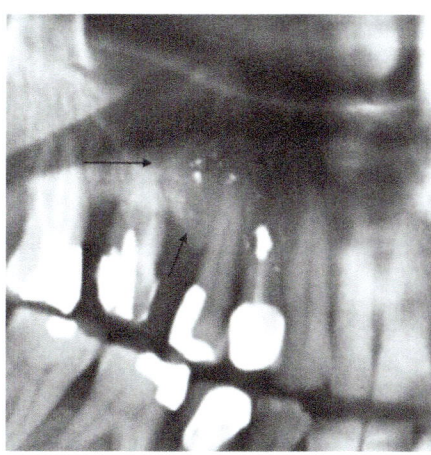

Fig. 8.19 Outflow of radiopaque material (indicated by *arrow*) towards the floor of the maxillary sinus

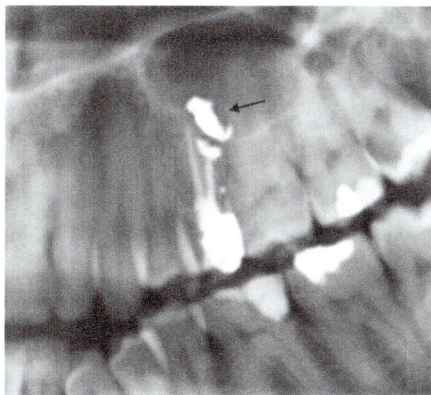

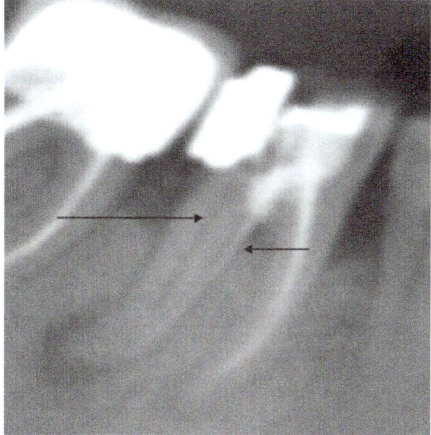

Fig. 8.20 False route with the presence of the filling material (indicated by *short arrow*) in the periodontal space. The dental canal (indicated by *long arrow*) appears not treated, and a periapical lesion is present

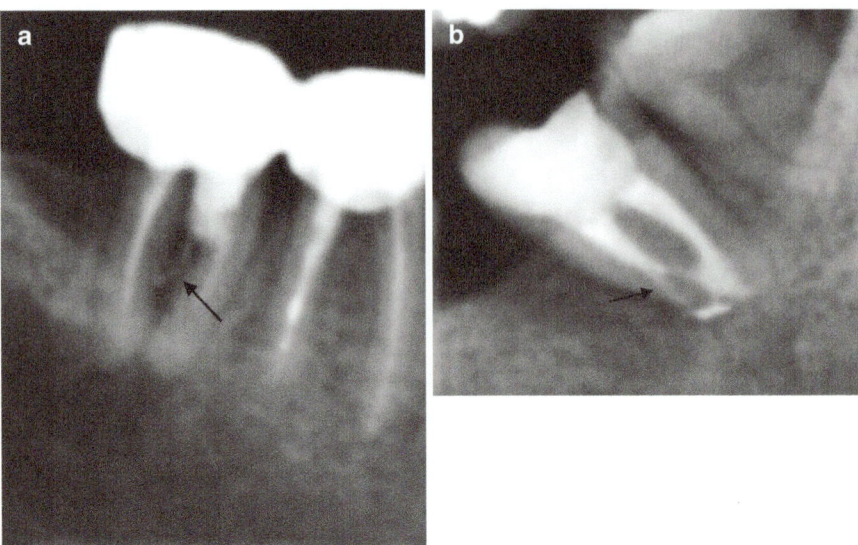

Fig. 8.21 (**a**, **b**) Small false routes (indicated by *arrows*) with poor clinical relevance

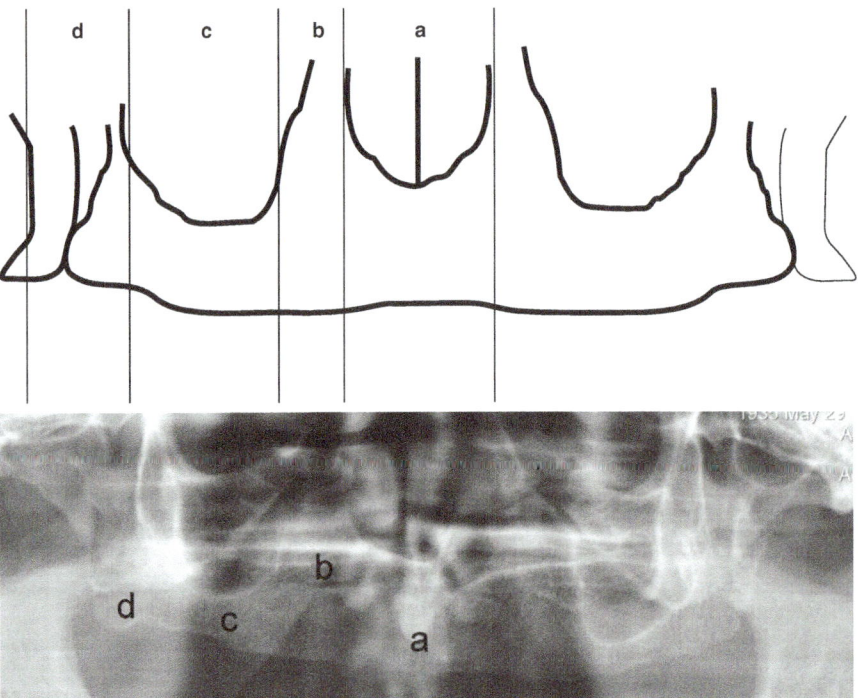

Fig. 8.22 Schematic diagram and radiographic representation of the subdivision of the superior maxillary based on the implantological perspective. (*a*) Central sector. (*b*) Canine pillar. (*c*) Subantral sector. (*d*) Maxillary tuberosity sector

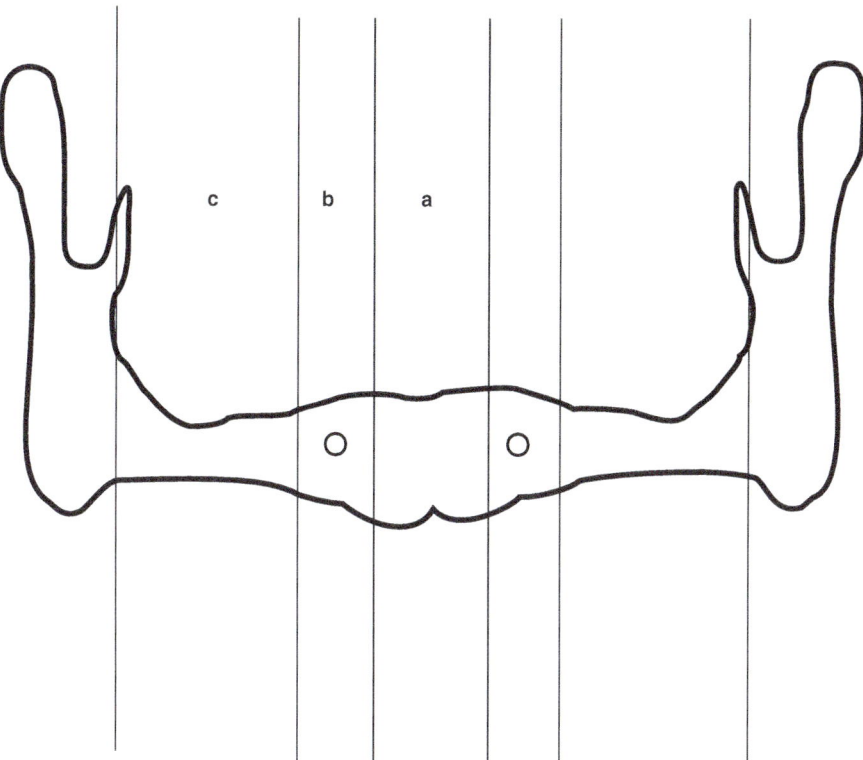

Fig. 8.23 Schematic diagram illustrating the subdivision of the inferior maxillary based on the implantological perspective. (*a*) Anterior sector. (*b*) Periforaminal sector. (*c*) Posterior sector

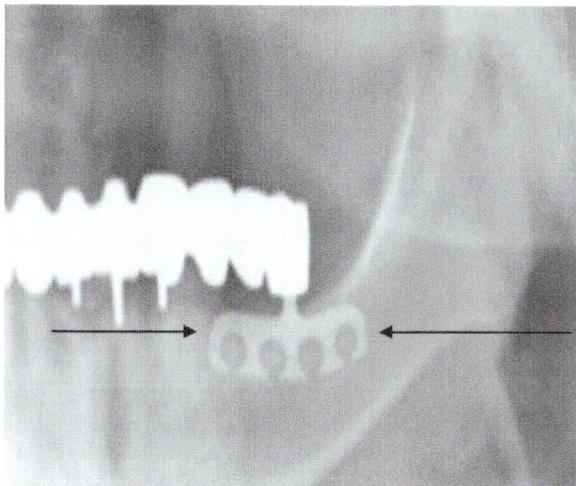

Fig. 8.24 Blade implant (indicated by *arrows*)

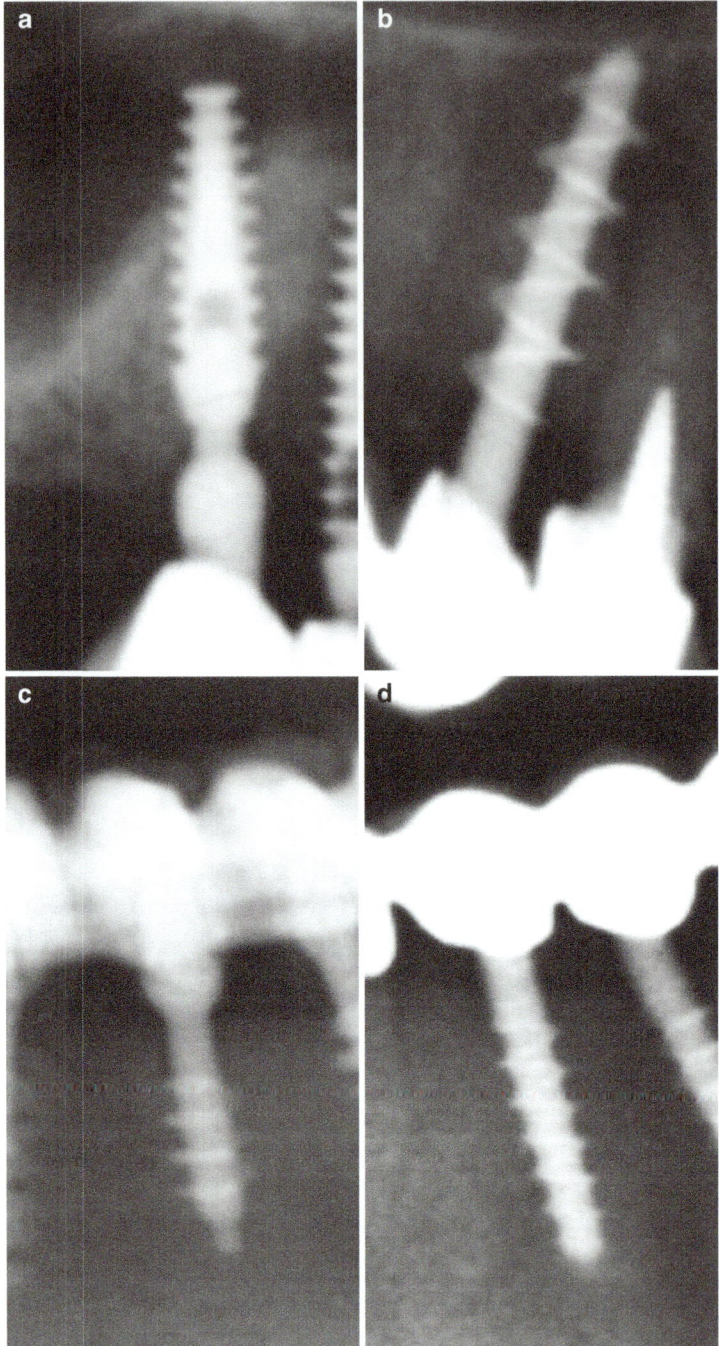

Fig. 8.25 (**a–d**) Different types of screw implants

Fig. 8.26 Implant device with cone morphology. (*1*) Neck. (*2*) Stem equipped with screw. (*3*) Closure screw

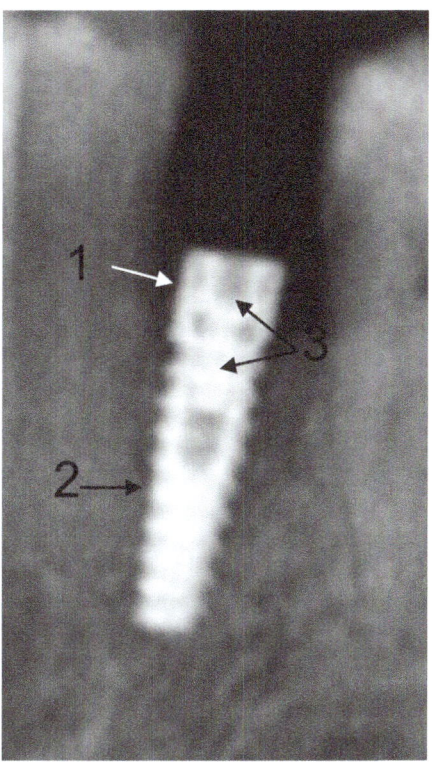

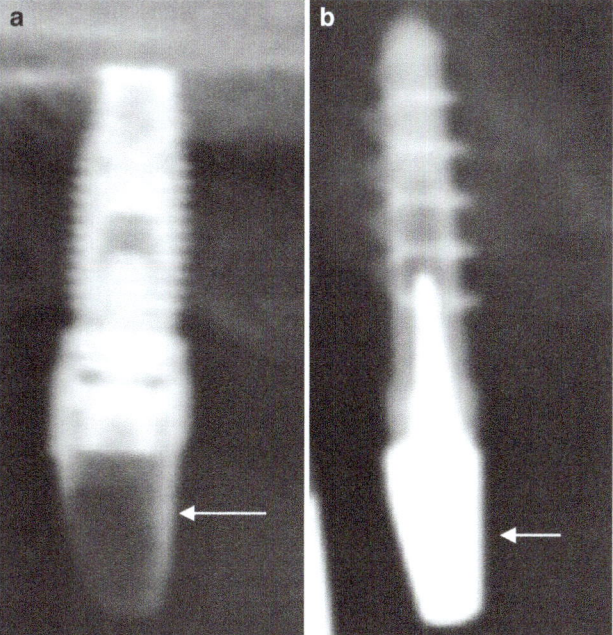

Fig. 8.27 (**a, b**) Two implant devices with different abutments (indicated by *arrows*)

Fig. 8.28 Complete implant procedure. (*1*) Implant device. (*2*) Abutment. (*3*) Crown prosthesis

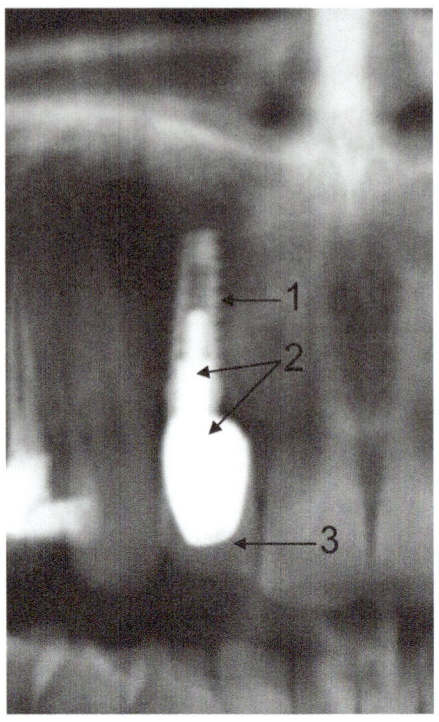

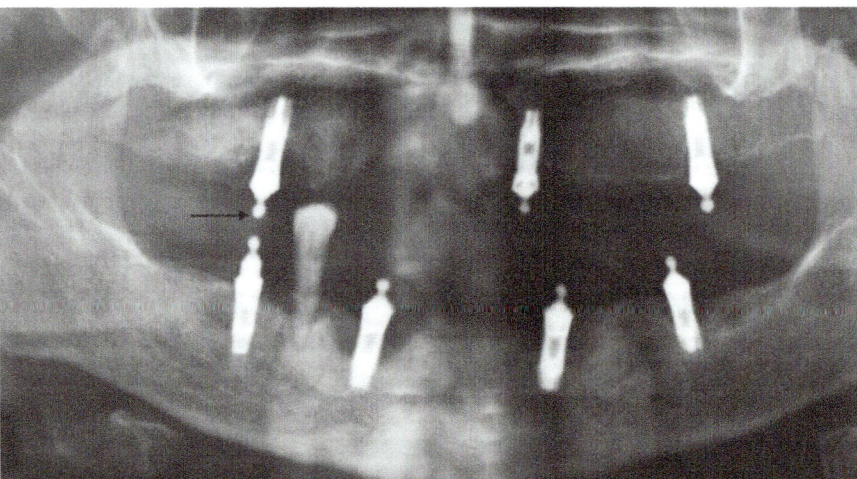

Fig. 8.29 Implants with abutments with spherical ending (indicated by *arrow*) for anchorage to mobile prosthesis

Fig. 8.30 Device for monophasic implant procedure

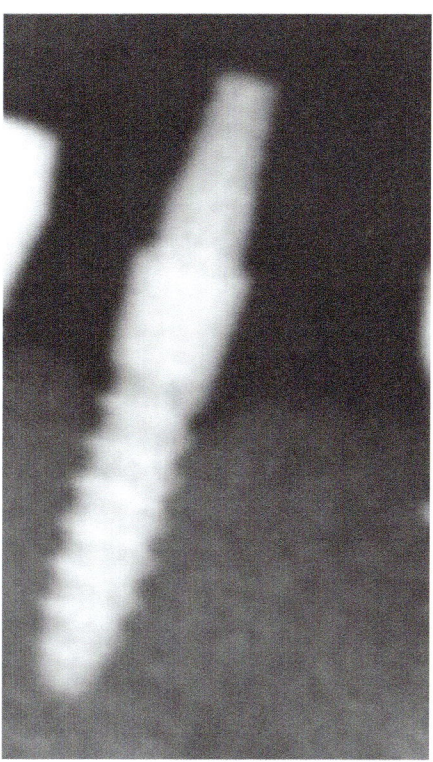

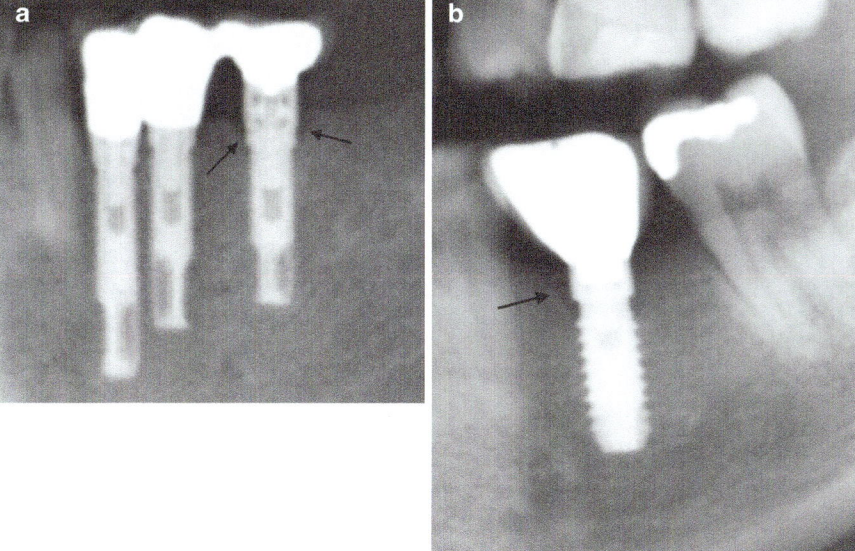

Fig. 8.31 Resorption cone of the bone adjacent to the neck (indicated by *arrows*). Both in (**a**, **b**) the phenomenon can be considered as physiologic

Fig. 8.32 Complete implant procedure with favourable crown/root ratio (see *arrows*)

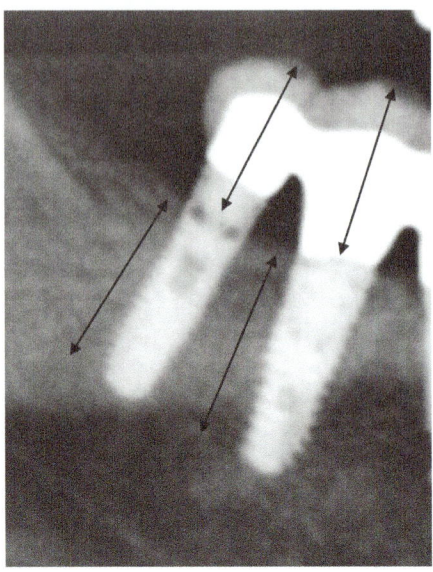

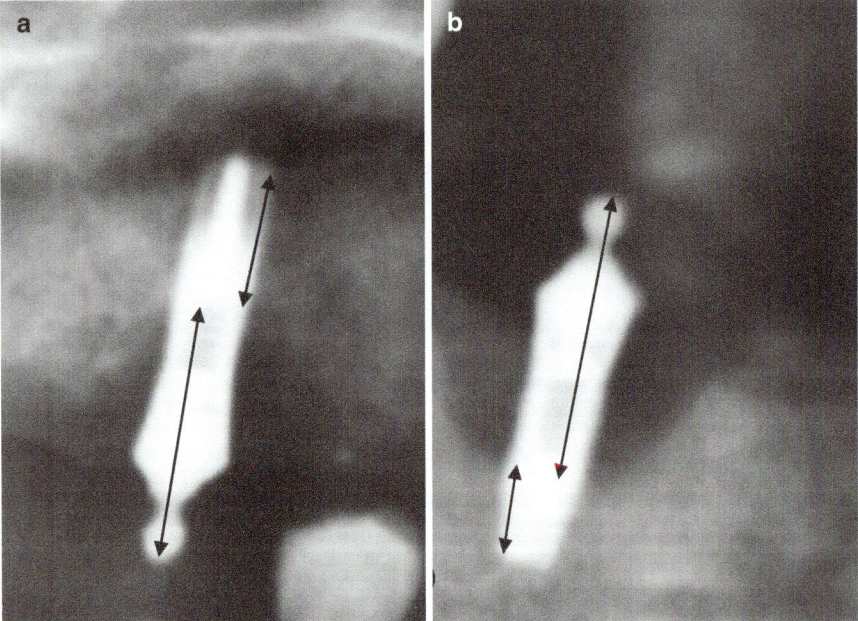

Fig. 8.33 (**a**) Shows critical crown/root ratio. (**b**) The crown/root ratio is reversed (see *arrows*)

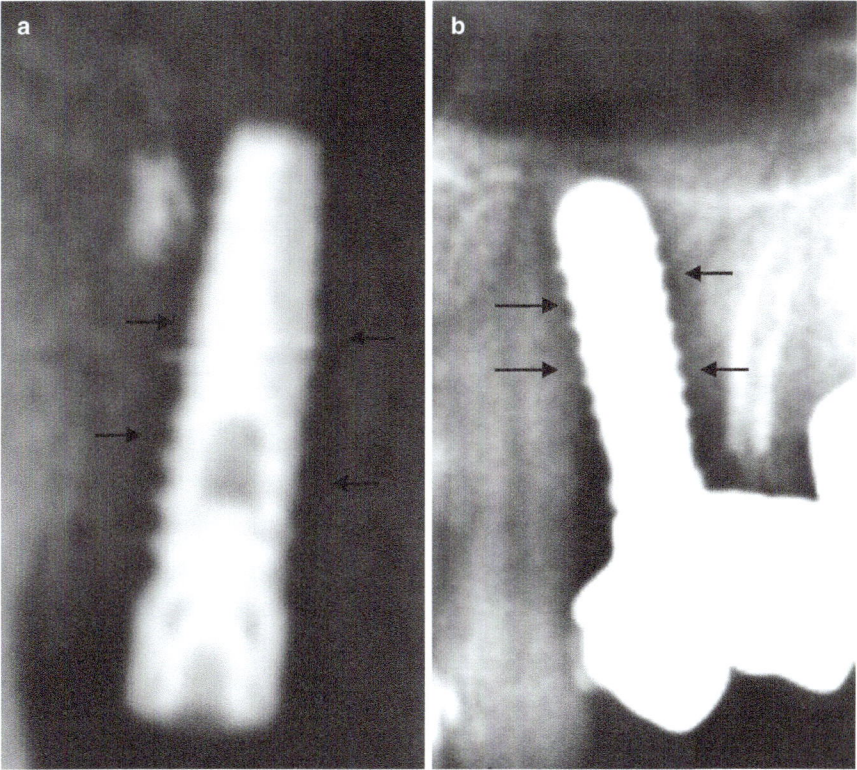

Fig. 8.34 (**a, b**) Two cases of very modest resorption bands of the peri-implant bone (indicated by *arrows*)

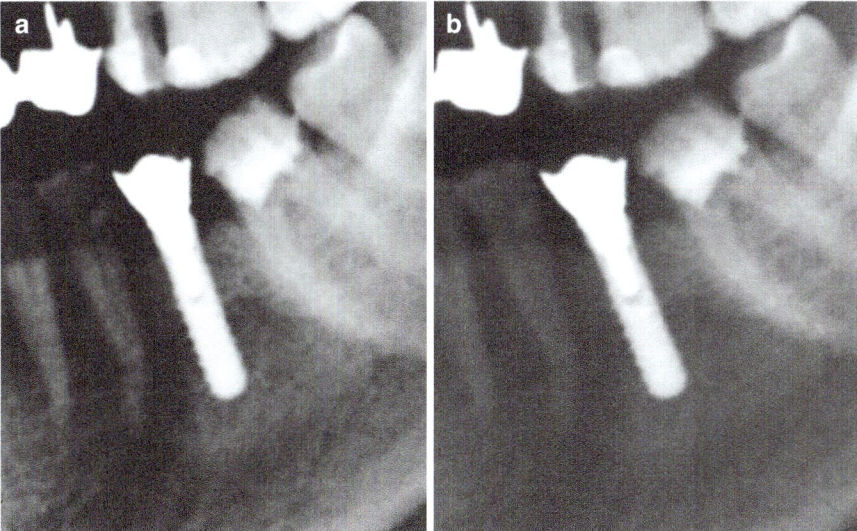

Fig. 8.35 (**a**) Digital reconstruction algorithm characterised by too strong edge enhancement effect can simulate the resorption of the peri-implant spongiosa. (**b**) Reconstruction with a more balanced algorithm showing the absolute normality of the peri-implant bone

Fig. 8.36 Blade implant with extended resorption process of the cancellous bone (indicated by *arrows*)

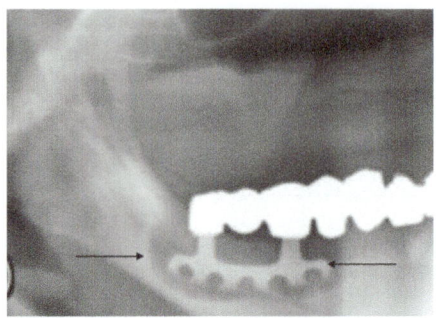

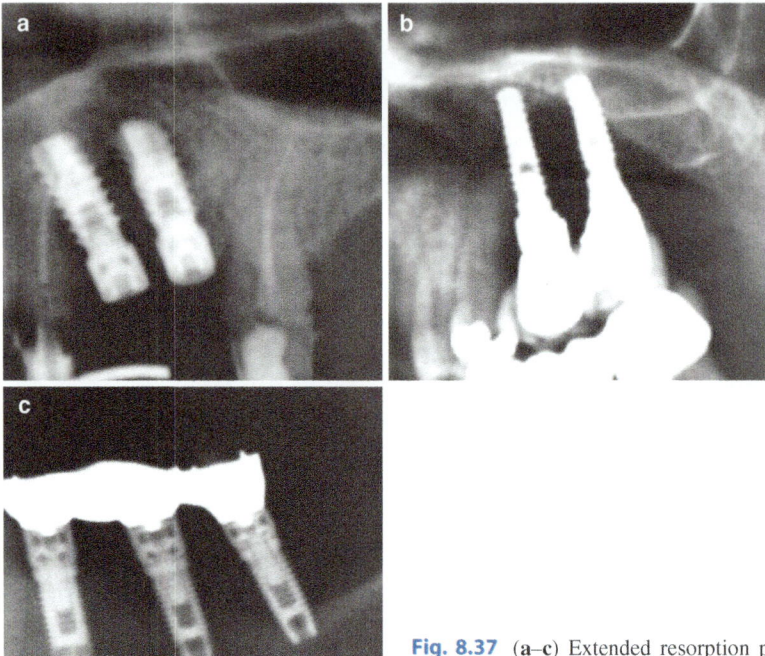

Fig. 8.37 (**a–c**) Extended resorption phenomena of the spongiosa with instable implants

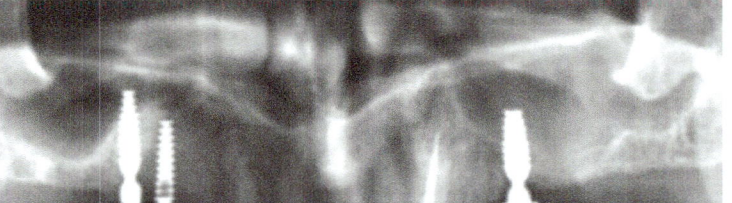

Fig. 8.38 On the right the implant apex is projected into the maxillary sinus which presents normal radiolucency. On the left the implant protrudes in the maxillary sinus which, conversely, is opacified

Fig. 8.39 Two implants (indicated by *long arrows*) protruding in the sinus wall with irregular thickness of the mucosa (indicated by *short arrows*)

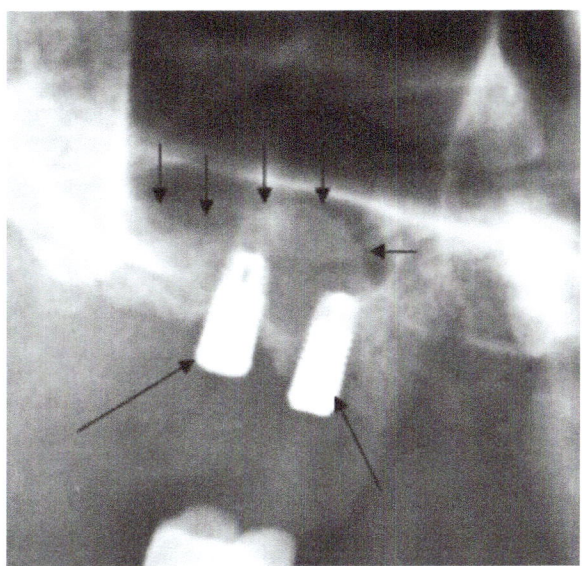

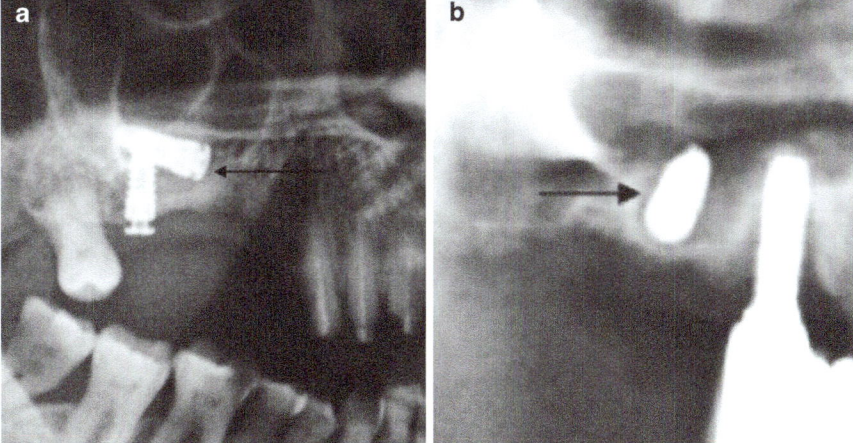

Fig. 8.40 (**a, b**) Two cases of implant devices (indicated by *arrows*) that have moved into the maxillary sinus

Fig. 8.41 Contact between the implant apex and the mental foramen (indicated by *arrow*). It is not possible to establish if real contact or a simple projective superimposition occurs

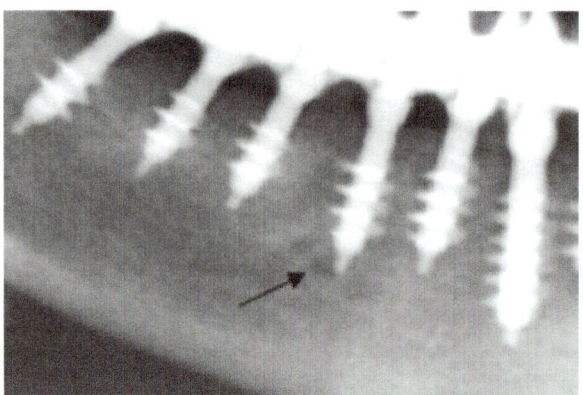

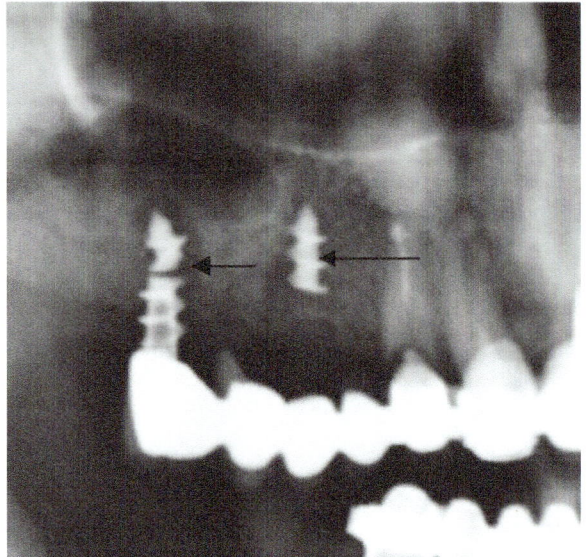

Fig. 8.42 Fracture of the implant in position 1.6 (indicated by *short arrow*). Implant fragment inclusive in the maxillary in position 1.4 (indicated by *long arrow*)

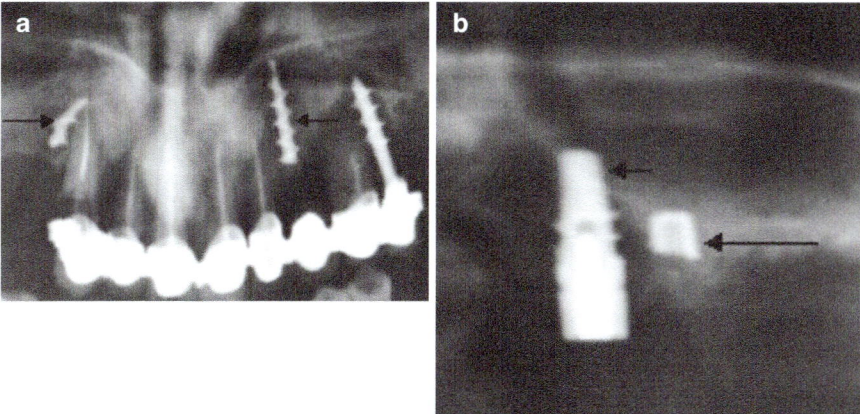

Fig. 8.43 (**a**, **b**) Two cases of residual implant fragments in the superior maxillary (indicated by *arrows*). The *short arrow* in (b) indicates the endosinusal protrusion of the implant apex

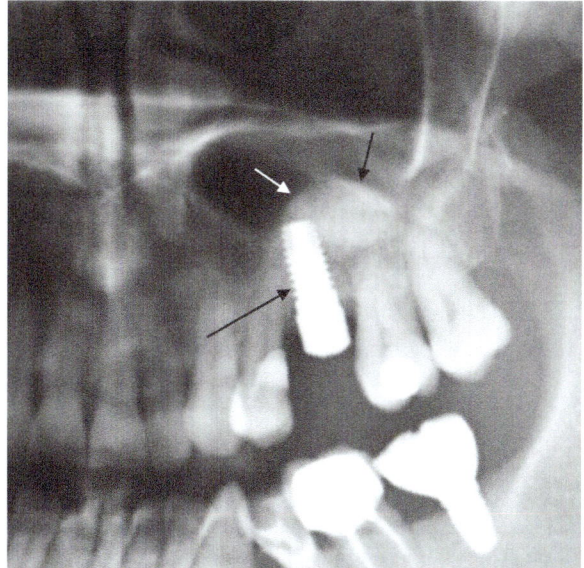

Fig. 8.44 Results of the left sinus floor augmentation (indicated by *short arrows*) which support a well-integrated implant (indicated by *long arrow*)

Suggested Reading

Abrahams JJ (1993) The role of diagnostic imaging in dental implantology. Radiol Clin North Am 31(1):163–180

Almong DM, Torrado E, Meitner SW (2001) Fabrication of imaging and surgical guides for dental implants. J Prosthet Dent 85(5):504–508

Basten CH (1995) The use of radiopaque templates for predictable implant placement. Quintessence Int 26(9):609–612

Benson BW (1995) Diagnostic imaging for dental implant assessment. Tex Dent J 112(2):37–41

Bouserhal G, Jacobs R, Quirynen M, Van Steenberghe D (2004) Imaging technique selection for the preoperative planning of oral implants: a review of literature. Clin Implant Dent Relat Res 4(3):156–172

Calgaro A, Bison L, Bellis GB, Pozzi Mucelli R (1999) Dentascan computed tomography of the mandibular incisive canal. Its radiologic anatomy and the therapeutic implications. Radiol Med 98(5):337–341

Chen LC, Lundgren T, Hallstrom H, Cherel F (2008) Comparison of different methods of assessing alveolar ridge dimensions to dental implant placement. J Periodontol 79(3):401–405

Danforth RA, Dus I, Mah J (2003) 3-D volume imaging for dentistry: an new dimension. J Calif Dent Assoc 31(11):817–823

De Smet E, Jacobs R, Gijbels F, Naert I (2002) The accuracy and reliability of radiographic methods for the assessment of marginal bone level around oral implants. Dentomaxillofac Radiol 31(3):176–181

Dula K, Mini R, Van der Stelt PF, Buser D (2001) The radiographic assessment of implant patients: decision making criteria. Int J Oral Maxillofac Implants 16(1):80–88

Garg AK, Vicari A (1995) Radiographic modalities for diagnosis and treatment planning in implant dentistry. Implant Soc 5(5):7–11

Gher ME, Richardson AC (1996) The accuracy of dental radiographic techniques used for evaluation of implant fixture placement. Int J Periodontics Restorative Dent 15(3):268–283

Jacobs R (2003) Preoperative radiologic planning of implant surgery in compromised patients. Periodontol 2000 33:12–25

Jeffcoat MK (1993) Application of digital radiography to implantology. J Dent Symp 1:30–33

Kassebaum DK, Stoller NH, Goshorn BI (1992) Radiographic techniques for presurgical assessment of dental implant sites. Gen Dent 40(6):502–5, 509–10

Kraut RA (1993) Effective uses radiographs for implant placements: panographs, cephalograms, CT scans. Dent Implantol Update 4(4):29–33

Lam EW, Ruprecht A, Yang J (1995) Comparison of two-dimensional orthoradially reformatted computed tomography and panoramic radiography for dental implant treatment planning. J Prosthet Dent 74(1):42–46

Lecomber AR, Yoneyama Y, Lovelock DJ, Hosoi T, Adams AM (2001) Comparison of patient dose from imaging protocols for dental implant planning using conventional radiography and computed tomography. Dentomaxillofac Radiol 30(5):255–259

Scribano E, Ascenti G, Mazziotti S, Blandino A, Racchiusa S, Gualniera P (2003) Computed tomography in dental implantology: medico-legal implications. Radiol Med 105(1–2):92–99

Index